Dogs

Are People, Too

Other books by Louis L. Vine, D. V. M.

Published in The United States:
   Common Sense Book of Complete Cat Care, Revised
Edition, 1992
   Your Neurotic Dog
   Total Dog Book
   Your Dog, His Health and Happiness (1974 Best Dog
Book of the Year)
   Dogs, Devils and Demons
   Behavior and Training of Puppies
   Breeding, Whelping and Natal Care of Dogs
   Dogs In My Life
Published abroad:
   Mon Chien A Des Problems, France
   Hunde Meine Liebsten Freunde, Germany
   Dogs Are My Patients, Great Britain
   Leilkibeteg Kutya, Hungary
   Vas Neuroticky Pes, Czechoslovakia

Dogs Are People, Too

(A Veterinarian's Memoire of Eccentric Dog Owners)

by

Louis L. Vine, D. V. M.

and

Greta Silver

Illustrations by
James Palmer

RIVERCROSS PUBLISHING, INC.
NEW YORK • ORLANDO

Printed in the United States of America. No part of this book may be used or reproduced in any manner whatsoever without written permission, except in the case of brief quotations embodied in critical articles and reviews. For information address RIVERCROSS PUBLISHING, INC., 127 East 59th Street, New York, NY 10022, or editor@rivercross.com

ISBN: 0-944957-66-8

Library of Congress Catalog Card Number: 97-1999

First Printing

Library of Congress Cataloging-in-Publication Data

Vine, Louis L.
    Dogs are people, too : a veterinarian's memoir of eccentric dog owners / by Louis L. Vine and Greta Silver ; illustrations by James Palmer.
        p.   cm.
    ISBN 0-944957-66-8
    1. Dogs—Anecdotes. 2. Dog owners—Anecdotes. 3. Vine, Louis L.
4. Veterinarians—North Carolina—Anecdotes. I. Silver, Greta.
II. Title.
SF426.2.V56   1997
636.7′088′7—dc21
                                                                        97-1999
                                                                        CIP

Table of Contents

Dedication:

This book is dedicated to all the thousands of my clients and their pets. Rest assured the names have been changed to protect the innocent . . . the dogs.

Introduction

During my 40 years as a veterinarian in Chapel Hill, North Carolina, I had many opportunities to observe the relationships between people and their dogs. As the years passed and increasing numbers of dog owners brought their animals to my clinic, it became more apparent that while there are as many variations of liaisons as there are breeds of dogs and varieties of people there were actually only two major types.

The first involved normal loving owners with well-trained dogs who responded immediately and correctly to their masters' glances, spoken commands or finger snaps. It didn't seem to matter whether owners of "good" pets instinctively knew how to train them, learned from their experience with past pets, or took them to obedience school for an elementary education in behavior. Nor did it matter whether these pets were pedigreed or mongrels. Nor was the coddled dog the happier one and, therefore, the best behaved pet on the block.

The more I spoke to people with obedient dogs, the more I realized that having pets who behaved well enough to delight Miss Manners depended to a great extent on the owners.

It helped if the human being in charge had the patience of Job, the wisdom of Solomon and the love of animals as Saint Francis of Assisi. And it really helped if that person also had eyes in the back of his head, was on the alert 24 hours a day and had what it took to care for a pet in all situations. Most of all, it helped if the owner were well-adjusted and acted normally around his or her dog. However, few people are endowed with all of these assets.

My clients with cooperative dogs tended to play down their own talents, intelligence and importance. They modestly felt their pets' behavior had nothing to do with the environment in which they lived, slept and ate and the amount of love, training and discipline they received. They gave all the credit to the "basically good" dogs. It was almost as if these animals had grown up by themselves, without human influence and determined how they wanted to turn out. This, of course, was not the case.

I came to realize that while these people considered their pets important and loving additions to their families, they distinguished clearly between two-legged and four-legged family members. People were people and dogs were dogs—nice owners with nice normal pets. And because the people were so normal, I don't vividly remember many of them today.

The owners I do remember clearly are those who have the second type of relationship—one that was unusual, sometimes extraordinary and often bizarre. In each combination of people and animals it was the owners—not the dogs—who behaved in ways that were comical, startling or outrageous. They were so unique that I began to allow more time between appointments to jot down their more spectacular stories and relate the dialogue between the owners and me as accurately as possible.

These people were overly enthralled by their dogs to the point where I considered them Dog-Gone. They were loving and apparently sensible, except when they were around their dogs. Then they invariably showed some degree of abnormal behavior.

About 99% of the time the problems rested with these owners who had an unusual definition of love. Thinking they were doing their pets a kindness, they humanized them until the dogs forgot how to be dogs and began to act like people. Yet, when I pointed this out to them they quickly argued, "Dogs are people, too."

When you talk to individuals who live with animals that were born dogs and still look, walk, sit and speak like dogs but are now considered and treated as people, you're bound to hear some mighty interesting stories.

I invite you to walk down memory lane with me to meet some of my most unforgettable characters. I suspect you'll never again look at a dog or its owner the way you do right now.

Chapter I

Average Dog Owners Versus Dog-Gone Owners

All dog owners look and act normal . . . like you and like me . . . until they're around their dogs.

Most owners talk to their dogs. When they say something particularly silly they might look around to see if anyone is listening. If so, it's common for them to defend themselves: "You have to admit that talking to my dog is more normal than talking to a flipping fern."

They don't worry about germs. They kiss their dog on the mouth immediately after he has finished licking himself. They justify this intimacy by saying, "Well, he might be a dog but his saliva is harmless because he's one of the family." That, any average dog owner knows, neutralizes all canine germs.

The average dog owner dearly loves his pet but usually puts people first. And because he believes in a well-defined distinction between people and dogs, he establishes and maintains

15

a role of dominance over his dog. This teaches pets that their owners are intolerant of and immune to canine manipulation. As a result of love tempered with discipline, the pets are usually very well trained.

When these people issue commands to their dogs they receive instant obedience. In rare instances, when their dogs ignore them, owners focus their attention on the dogs, reprimand them, reissue the command and make sure they carry through. At times like this, they have been known to say, "Dammit, Jake, stop it. Remember I'm the person and you're the dog." (See illustration 1.)

In a nutshell, average dog owners are so normal and predictable they're downright boring. So let's get to the good stuff.

Dog-Gone Owners couldn't care less who hears them talk to their dogs, even when they're talking baby talk or complete nonsense. They feel there's absolutely no need to make excuses when it's written in drool that dogs listen better, understand more and communicate more clearly than people.

As far as kissy poo goes, these owners realize there's no need to worry about neutralizing canine germs as they are non-existent. On the contrary, people should worry about passing on their own filthy killer germs and viruses to their dogs.

"Actually," says one owner who considers herself quite knowledgeable, "you can and do get more germs from kissing people. Dog kisses are quite harmless compared to those of humans. You should tell people that a dog's kiss has healing power because the strong enzymes in the saliva are cleansing and curative."

Dog-Gone Owners generally love their pets more than people. Even if they don't, they tend to put their pets first. Also,

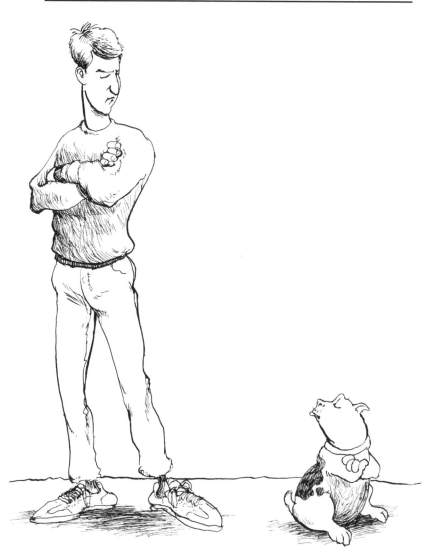

1. Who's the boss

they rarely consider their own needs first. The distinction between these mortals and their pets is fuzzy, and tends to create owners who constantly transmit messages that they are submissive to the boss dogs. This often creates demanding and manipulative pets. As a result, these owners are usually very well trained. (See illustration 2.)

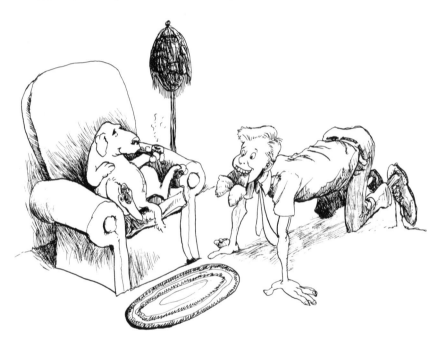

2. Dog domination

When they issue commands to their dogs they're often accompanied by a "que sera, sera" attitude. One owner was quoted as saying, "Mother, Obie doesn't feel like getting off the chair now, so prop your cane in the corner and pull up another chair."

You have to understand these owners. They just cannot hide the fact that they've allowed their pets to consume their lives, hearts and common sense. You might be looking at a dog, but they are not. They're looking at sons, daughters, friends or lovers. Those pedigrees or mutts are people. At times they can also be confidantes, gurus, lovers in a spiritual or Biblical sense, or the reincarnation of a departed loved one.

Some of these dogs are even considered extensions of Dog-Gone Owners as evinced by remarks such as, "We aren't feeling well, today," and "Our laxative just kicked in. Let's go potty."

They live by the conviction, "Love me, love my dog." The LMLMD principle makes perfect sense to them. They assume that if you care about them, you will realize how very much they love their dogs and, therefore, you, will love them too. If you don't, then there's something wrong with you.

(See illustration 3.)

This can be a lot of medicine to swallow if you're not a dog lover, or even if you are an average dog owner who just insists on good manners from your pets. When you see these Dog-Gone Owners in action, and hear what they have to say, you'll probably doubt that you actually saw or heard what you know you saw or heard.

Here's an example that boggled my mind 32 years ago. One of my clients told me she dressed her dog for beddy-bye in shortie nighties with matching panties. (Don't forget, dogs are people, too, and people generally wear bed clothes.) Once the dog was properly attired, she put Sapphire into her doggy bed, read her a story and kissed her goodnight. This nightly ritual went on for 12 years until Sapphire passed on.

Dog-Gone Owners may not get down on all fours to lap water out of the bowl on the floor, at least not in front of you, but they do over-identify with their dogs. The extent of their

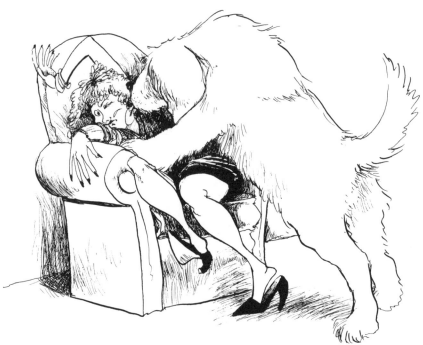

3. Social climber

unusual behavior can range from "a tad loco" to "in a million years you wouldn't believe." While they are all not extreme, this group contains a large number who encourage craziness in their dogs. In fact, they are the number one reason 10% of dogs show some signs of abnormal behavior.

How do you know if a relative, friend or acquaintance is going to be an average dog owner or a Dog-Gone Owner? You can bet your life savings you won't know until they're holding the leash.

Psychologists have touched on the subject of people and pets, but they have not analyzed or compared a wide range of dog owners. The experts merely point out that a person's choice of a dog reveals his idiosyncrasies, character defects, weaknesses, needs and desires. This theory has given birth to a lot of stereotypes you've heard many times. Some of the most popular ones are:

Meek people choose large aggressive dogs to compensate for what they lack.

Angry people who want to bully and dominate others choose large dogs to transform them into macho men or ma-cha mommas.

High-strung individuals choose hyperactive dogs. (See illustration 4.)

Small men choose large dogs to make them feel macho. (See illustration 5.)

People choose pets that resemble them. (See illustration 6.)

The list goes on and on. Let's say that these generalizations are occasionally correct. Most often they aren't, yet people who don't have dogs tend to believe them.

Dog owners, however, thumb their noses at the experts and theories, and say, "What a pile of poop!" Equally remiss as psychologists, they sum up dog owners by saying that a person's choice of a dog reveals his common sense, trust, love, good character, eagerness for responsibility and sense of humor.

To both schools I say, "Get out the scooper."

Here's what I learned from my clients: In every group of people, and dog owners are no exception, you'll find saints, sweethearts, sadists and stinkers. You'll find healthy people and not so healthy people, sane and not so sane, good and bad—contrasts all the way down the line. How do you know who's who and what kind of dog owner he or she will be after being handed the leash? You don't. Most importantly, how

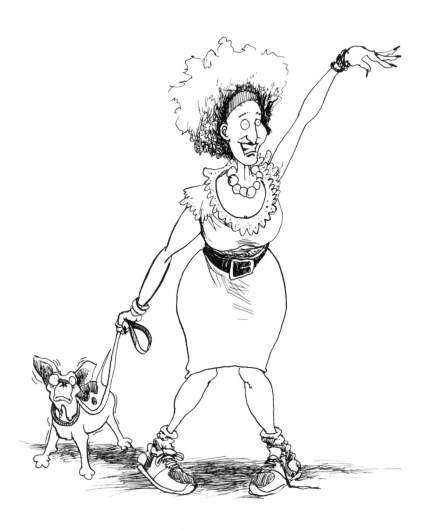

4. *Like master—like dog*

do you know which owners will turn out to be average and which have the makings of Dog-Gone Owners? You don't.

When I questioned my clients on their choice of dogs, most told me that they didn't know what they were looking for when they went shopping. They rarely took their own personalities into consideration, never counted how many jokes they cracked per day, and gave little or no thought to the type of dog owner they'd be. They just decided to get a dog. Period.

Perhaps a small percentage of them preferred one breed. Most folks, however, decided beforehand whether they wanted a small dog, big dog, sweet dog, watch dog, patient and tolerant dog, long-haired or short-haired dog, seeing eye dog, or a dog to take the place of dear departed Dufus. That's where their conscious thinking ended before they went into action and actually found a dog.

Choosing the dog almost always depended on rapport between the two.

It was a good, better or best decision based on logical, illogical or no thought, and it was the decision they intuitively acknowledged. At the very least, it was positive enough for them to decide on the spot, "That's the ideal doggy for me!"

More than once I've bemoaned the fact that anybody, even a Marquis de Sade, can own a dog. The license to buy or adopt hinges merely on three words: "I want one." Why do they want one? "Just 'cause." All too often less thought is given to owning a pet that will share a household for 10 to 15 years than to buying a pair of athletic shoes that last one season.

There should be some way of pre-screening prospective owners to determine if they're capable and responsible enough to be entrusted with pets. Nothing radical, mind you, just a method that quickly and painlessly allows a person like Solomon or Judge Wapner to evaluate a person before he renders his verdict. Or, let the dogs decide. Let them point paw up or paw down and determine their fate rather than be at the mercy of characters we wouldn't want to be related to.

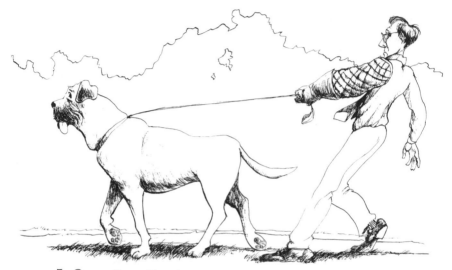

5. Opposites attract

After dealing with thousands of clients, I'm convinced there's no accurate barometer that foretells whether a person will be a good or poor, average owner or exceptional owner. You know only after the fact, when you see a person/dog duo relating and interacting.

If you see yourself in any of the following chapters, you can betcha bow-wow you have the makings of a Dog-Gone Owner. Or, perhaps you're already one. But relax, because you'll never equal Francis Henry Egerton, the eighth Earl of Bridgewater who lived in the 19th century.

Sir Francis was a lonely man who had difficulty relating to people. Preferring the company of dogs, he regularly took six of them along when he went for carriage rides. The townfolk talked about that almost as much as they gossiped about his reported passion for footwear.

Luckily Sir Francis had the money and closet space to indulge in different boots or shoes 365 days a year. Some of his less fortunate neighbors had a few things to say about his fetish because it extended to the canine friends he also outfitted in fine leather boots. The topper to his Dog-Gone hall of fame, however, were the parties he hosted.

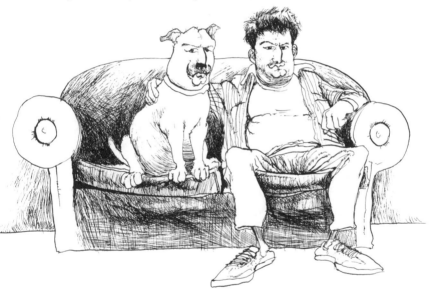

6. Dog and people look-alikes

When Sir Francis was in a festive mood he'd have his servants set the table for 12 with damask, china, crystal and sterling. Then his favorite dogs, all dressed in the height of dog fashion, were escorted in by personal servants to the dining room chairs. After tying a napkin around the neck of his charge, each servant served his charge extraordinary gourmet delights. While the dogs nibbled at or wolfed down their meals, Sir Francis conversed with them. According to one blabbermouth servant, the typical conversation went something like this:

"How is the filet mignon, friends?"

"Grrrreat!"

"So, how was your day, Fluffy?"

"Ruff!"

"Seconds, Duchess?"

"Yip."

All right, Sir Francis was a bit eccentric. But you have to admire his individuality and the fact that he didn't care what anyone thought of him. He did what he wanted, benefitting himself and his lucky pets until they died before their time . .

thanks to gross obesity.

Remember that what I'm about to say is only my opinion, including personal biases and observations over a period of four decades. A mere 40 years, folks. You might not agree with some of my conclusions, but that's all right. Not everyone buys chicken-flavored dog food. That's why there are beef, liver and veal flavors, too.

Chapter 2

The Food Bowl Runneth Over

When Wendy brought her puppy in for a checkup she was concerned enough about her pet's development to follow my feeding suggestions. The same can be said for all my clients with puppies, from Abigail to Zoe and Amery to Zachary. It was easy for them to agree because they saw instant results of full, distended bellies after every meal. That indicated to them that their pets were properly fed, healthy and thriving. The chubbier the puppy, the happier the owner.

Then the pups grew up, naturally slimmed down and their dietary requirements changed. It was at this point that I explained to clients that what went in the dog was as important as what came out.

"Picture a scale of justice with both sides perfectly balanced with dog food on one side and your dog's bowel movement on the other. The proper food in the proper amount results in healthy elimination. That's balance. That's what you should think of when it comes to your pet's diet. If you feed your dog too much or you feed him improper food, it tips the scale. You'll end up with a fat dog, or a dog with digestive problems. You wouldn't want that, would you?"

Knowing that clients would agree to anything just to get away from the unappetizing picture I presented, I'd close with the clincher. "Now in order to keep that scale balanced I recommend the ideal canine diet of water and nourishing dog food."

Most dog owners took this suggestion in stride, commenting it was easy, convenient and eliminated the guess work for them. "Besides," many said, "I realize it's the best food for my dog." When clients reacted this way I knew dog food would be the mainstay of Fergie's or Fritzie's diet . . . except for the daily treats they managed to scrounge from sympathetic family members. All in all, though, a sensible diet.

However, many Dog-Gone Owners, especially those who were overweight, had difficulty digesting the unpalatable news that commercial dog food was the way to go. That thinking makes sense if you look at it from their point of view. Their dog, a person, should be like other people who love to eat favorite and different items at each meal and different meals each day. No matter how they tried, they could not fit dog food into an edible category.

It must have seemed like skid row fare when they compared it to the steak and potatoes, shrimp scampi and rice, burgers and fries, and the multitude of other mouth watering delicacies they ate. Even the thought of their dog drinking tap water to wash down the glop while they sipped their beverages of choice had to seem inhuman except to those few who believe water is life's elixir.

One client paled and gasped, "Oh, no!" and placed her hand over her heart as if I had shocked her. "Dog food? We're talking about Bootsie!" Most clients didn't over-react that much. After saying, "How boring!" they'd hesitantly agree to go along with dog food "temporarily to see if he survives."

"Dogs don't mind," I told them. "A dog thinks he's getting a feast if he gets the same dry or canned dog food everyday. If you want him to think he's getting gourmet food, mix the dry and the canned dog food together. Believe me, your pet won't get tired of it."

Barry disagreed. "Come off it, Doc," he said. "You'd get tired of filet mignon if you had to eat it every night for the rest of your life. You couldn't. You'd want change."

Barry and I argued about change whenever we met. "Gruff wants different dog food to chomp into." "He's tired of the same junk." "He told me he's going on an eating strike." In fact, Gruff was content with his uninspired diet; it was Barry who was having a hard time tolerating it.

Then he left Gruff with a friend and he went away for three days. He called when he returned. "Remember I told you Gruff was going to go on an eating strike? He did. He didn't eat a bit the whole time I was gone."

"That's not unusual when a dog has a strong bond with his master," I told him. "He missed you."

"When I got home I fed him his regular stuff. He only ate a little bit, not his usual two cans."

"Not unusual. He was letting you know he was angry you had left him."

"The next day I gave him two cans of new stuff. He loved it and then he walked over to me and puked."

"Not unusual, he . . . "

"For Chrissake, stop saying 'not unusual!' What I'm trying to tell you is that he has been getting worse every day. He throws up after every meal and has diarrhea all over the house. I think he's dying!"

"All right, Barry, I hear you. Now listen . . . "

"He's dying!" he repeated frantically. "I never should have left him. It's all my fault."

I didn't know whether to feel sorrier for Barry or Gruff. Gruff might have been a big dog, but similar to most he had a delicate digestive system. He couldn't tolerate a feast, especially since it had abruptly replaced his regular fare. The dog made an amazing recovery when he ate his old food, and Barry changed his mind about change.

"Never again," he said.

"That's a relief."

"Yeah, I'm never going to leave Gruff alone again. And the next time I know he's bored out of his mind from his food I'll just add a little bit of the new stuff."

To my knowledge, the only concerned owner who didn't share the variety is the spice of life belief is a college chum who is completely uninterested in food. Matt literally lived on vegetable pizza and cola for breakfast, lunch and dinner. He, I'm sure, appreciated the idea of unvaried dog meals. But most Dog-Gone clients who imagined themselves limited to one food item and one beverage for the rest of their lives compared it to torture for pets.

"I'd slash my wrists!" one woman insisted.

She was just as unhappy as the gentleman who tried to convince me that monotonous meals kill a dog's taste buds.

"How's that?" I asked Tom.

"All dog foods look the same, smell the same, and have the same texture and color. What's the difference? Crunchy stuff or mushy stuff. Even if they're mixed, the dog knows he's going to get the same garbage. There's no excitement, no anticipation, no gusto. He just piles it in, shoves it around, chews it a couple of times and swallows it. So his taste buds aren't challenged. They go to sleep, fall into a coma and die."

"That's an interesting theory but it doesn't change my thinking." I was more adamant six months later when Tom brought in Itsy Bitsy, the blimp. "I see that your cocker's taste buds lived," I told him. "She's seven pounds overweight. That's the equivalent of 40 pounds on you!" After swearing that Itsy Bitsy must have blown up from inhaling crumbs that fell on the floor . . . "and she must be allergic to them" . . . Tom admitted the family supplemented her dog food with table scraps and handouts sneaked under the table. "And, she has to have buttered popcorn at night when we watch TV."

Determined clients who wanted to show me the way brought up the dog's diet over and over again. Once I became so annoyed rehashing the kibble bit that I yelled, "Gladys, raise your right hand and swear you'll feed Mopsy dog food and nothing but dog food, so help you God!"

"I can't because I won't. But I'll try."

Each conference ended with owners grudgingly agreeing to follow my instructions, while both of us knew they'd do exactly what they wanted to do. Usually, they tipped me off to their plans before they left the clinic. One no-nonsense guy, said, "Hey, Doc, only a moron eats the same stuff every day and Brutus isn't a moron." Most were a bit more subtle, and took the back door approach to warn me.

"I've been thinking that a few tablespoons of people food can't hurt Mooch if it's mixed in with a lot of dog food." Or . . .

"I'll cut Scooter's table scraps in half." Or . . .

"It breaks my heart to see Diablo beg when we're eating."

Judging by the love handles on the pets' hips I venture to say that 99% continued to relish more than their fair share. Around 50% to 60% of my patients were overweight, ranging from borderline to grossly obese, and too many were proportionally as pudgy as their owners. (See illustration 7.)

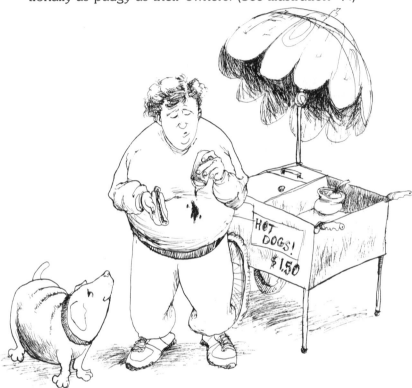

7. Fat People—fat dog

As a veterinarian I enjoyed seeing slim dogs as much as doctors like to see slim people. I can't count the times I felt like baying at the moon seeing yet another obese dog waddle in and pant for breath. Yet, while the majority of my clients celebrated when they lost a few pounds, these same owners panicked if they suspected their chunky pets had lost an ounce or two. On the other hand, there is a health-conscious client who maintains a near perfect body weight by watching his own diet carefully, but who gives all the extra high caloric food to his obese dog. It's obvious that dogs are at the mercy of their owner's whims. (See illustration #8)

One client was sure Scottie Fenster was ailing. "Look at him," insisted Lucy. "He's all bones. His ribs stick out. I hope he doesn't have a tumor or tape worms." As it turned out, Fenster was in ideal condition. He was simply an active, healthy dog.

Despite my reassurances, Lucy decided she knew something was wrong. I may have been the vet, but according to her I had not pinpointed a problem she intuitively knew existed. It took a lot of reassuring on my part and blood tests for the dog for her to relax. Even then, Lucy suggested I add a supplement like Ensure to Fenster's meals. "A special dog needs a special diet."

While we're on the subject of special diets, let's discuss three exceptional ones I came across.

One little old lady fed her German Shepherd only chocolate covered peanuts. Nothing else. She had a very logical reason. "I did research and it proved that every necessary nutrient Hans needs are in peanuts." Therefore, she hand fed him peanut after peanut every day of his life. Nothing I said deterred her from this unique diet. Hans seemed fine . . . except for needing an enema once a month.

Zeb brought in a large hound dog who was not very happy to see me. Zeb wrapped his hands and arms around the dog, and pinned him down with his chest to keep Masher on the table, telling me between Masher's growls, snarls and bared fangs that "He don't like strangers much . . . he's one son-of-a bitchin' mean dog." I called in an assistant to hold Masher's head so I could examine his mouth and teeth.

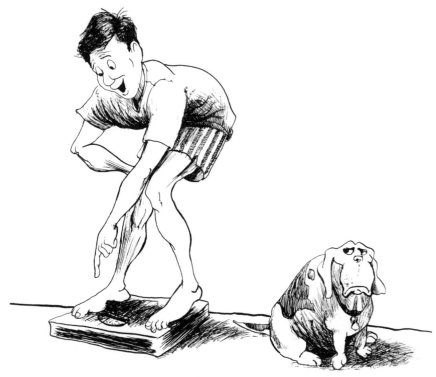

8. Man's best diet friend

"The reason we're here," Zeb said, "is Masher burps like crazy. Can't understand why." Just then Masher let loose a ripper of a belch, and for an encore produced a commendable salvo of short repeats.

We got around to the subject of diet and that's when I heard about feeding a dog gunpowder steak tartar, meat seasoned with gunpowder, to make him mean and aggressive. Maybe you've heard this old wive's tale but I wasn't aware of it until then.

I was worried that Masher would self destruct, so I called another country client to ask what he fed his dogs.

"Meat and gunpowder," he said, as if it was the most ordinary dog diet in the world. "It isn't harmful, Doc, but it does give a dog an explosive nature."

Finally, there was the naturalist who lived off the land. He neither wanted to worry about his dog's diet or foul the environment. In this interest, and because he believed wholeheartedly in recycling, he fed his dog nothing but horse manure.

"Horse shit. He loves it," owner Cliff said, "especially if it's right out of the oven. And it sure is because I bought two horses so he has a fresh supply every day." I asked how long Snaps had been a manure muncher. "Two years," he told me. After examining the mutt I found him to be in excellent health. He did, however, require charcoal tablets because he had one hell of a case of halitosis.

These three clients differed radically from the Dog-Gone Owners who fed their pets the same or better foods than they consumed. The majority managed to do this without "slaving over a hot stove." They opened a package or can of dog food, emptied the contents into the dog's feeding bowl, and mixed in "just a touch of bacon fat" or other delicacy to make the food more palatable. Those who felt "everyone needs hot meals" went one step farther by heating the food in a microwave or on the stove top. However, approximately 30% of dog owners relied solely on commercial baby foods, rationalizing, "Well, he is my baby!"

"Baby food is fine as an occasional treat for Blue," I told a client whose dog wouldn't know dog grub if she fell over it. "Sometimes I even recommend it for a dog with a digestive upset or a chronic gastric problem. Blue does not need it."

"She tells me she loves Gerbers. It goes down easily."

"Right. But junior foods don't give her much to chew and it doesn't give her teeth or gums any exercise. That's why she's having dental problems."

"What should we do?"

"Switch her over to dog food."

"Dog food? It's horrid! You've got to be out of your mind!"

Once in a great while a dog refused to eat people food. One of the smartest dogs I knew turned up his nose in disgust when his owner offered him a burger from a famous franchise. "There must be something wrong with him. We can't get enough of them. And Lickety actually prefers dog food," she said in amazement. "I wish he had a better sense of taste."

However, given the choice, most dogs opted for the same foods their owners ate. For example, twice a week Perky's mom felt guilty that she arrived home late from work, and made amends by buying him a McDonalds burger. "He knows when it's Tuesdays and Thursdays," she told me. "He greets me at the door, holding his food bowl between his teeth. The other days he doesn't bother to bring me his bowl." (See illustration 9)

"He's a smart pup," I replied.

"Smart? He's brilliant," she said. And then quite seriously, she said, "I wish there were Mensa tests for dogs. I'm sure he's a genius. After all, he paws off the top of the bun, picks out the pickle slices and the lettuce and gives them to me to eat."

But had Dog-Gone Owners tasted a few of the canned products they would have been surprised to discover that it was not all that bad. "It reminds me of pate," said one adventurous client.

One gentleman agreed. His ex-wife was scheduled to come to his house to return a brooch his mother had given her. Still stinging from the ugly divorce, he didn't feel as generous and

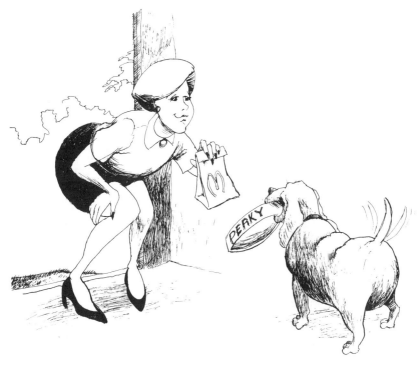

9. Perky's burger

forgiving as she. "That witch made me give up my dog because she said Punky stunk up the house, and how could she
have her friends or culinary club come to the house when it
was her turn to cook a fancy schmancy meal."

He invited her to have a drink and snacks. Much to his glee,
she accepted. He offered her a strong martini, and canapes
of mashed dog food on crackers with a pimiento garnish that
he had artfully arranged on a plate. "Let me tell you it was
the best thing I did for myself since the divorce. She almost
went nuts trying to identify the ingredients of the spread, said

it had an 'interesting and different' taste, and asked for the recipe. I told her I had sworn on my grandmother's death bed never to reveal her secret."

That reminds me of a sad story. One of my clients told me that her husband, Henry, loved to eat canned dog food and consumed many cases of it before he met an untimely end. He was killed while chasing cars down the street. I swear I'm telling the truth.

When I asked the widow why Henry developed an affinity for canned dog food, she replied, "It all happened because our poodle Tinkle wouldn't eat her food unless one of us tasted and chewed it first. Since I have a weak stomach, Henry did it. Before long, he was eating more of the dog food than little Tinkle. I believe Henry actually began to think like a dog, and he started to chase cars. You know the rest. I haven't been the same since."

"I can believe it," I said.

Dog food manufacturers realize dogs are big business. They also know that people, not dogs, buy their foodstuffs. In order to encourage owners of dogs with picky palates to purchase their products, they've attempted to improve the quality over the years. They've succeeded very well.

There's virtually a smorgasbord of available dog food at the local food market or pet store—more than enough to satisfy any Dog-Gone Owner. The flavor is right, the consistency is fine, and the smell is acceptable. Some mimic the tastes of human foods so well they could fool an inebriated late night snacker who craves some left-over meatballs.

There are high protein foods for the growing puppy and low calorie foods for the dog who wants to keep a "youthful" figure. There are geriatric formulas for the senior citizens and hypoallergenic choices for sensitive dogs. And there are organic foods for health-minded canines, as well as ethnic delights for dogs of different cultural backgrounds and religions.

You name it, it's available. (An interesting aside is that in 1976 one manufacturer tested a birth control canned dog food to inhibit bitches from coming into heat. To my knowledge it did not take off. That's not to say it won't become available eventually.)

One enterprising dog food company specializing in ethnic dog foods has a gourmet Italian style food consisting mainly of beef or chicken and pasta in a tomato based sauce. It is made with pure olive oil. Take your choice of Bolognese or Cacciatore. Frankly, it looks and smells very good. Being a lover of Italian food, I'm more and more tempted to try it.

The company also offers Kosher style canned food for Jewish dogs who wish to adhere to a strict dietary code. True to orthodox Jewish laws, dairy and meat products are not mixed. They have a meat style food and also a dairy product food that includes cheeses and vegetables. Absolutely no pork by-products are used in their meat canned food. Heaven forbid!

Another type of canned food is an Irish stew with plenty of beef and vegetables. And for the oriental breeds, such as the Char-pei, there's a chop suey mixture.

Ordinary dog food is tasty enough for about 20% of the human population who are on limited budgets, or have exotic tastes like Henry, or who have adventurous souls. If dog food companies make their foods any more delectable, I'll be eating my poodle's food. Yet, judging by the millions of Dog-Gone Owners who cannot be convinced to buy it, it's not good enough for dogs.

Lucky for them more specialty stores are opening around the country each year. One franchise operation, the Puppy Hut, founded in Toledo, Ohio has branches in Chicago, Detroit, Miami, Orlando and Pittsburgh. The successful business is a doggy delight, complete with a drive-thru widow, "Park and Bark" picnic area and fire hydrant. Dog owners are willing to pay a bit more than they would for dog treats at the supermarket because they get pleasure seeing their pets munch, socialize and sniff each other, and cavort around the hydrant.

However, if owners consider picnics a bit too informal and loathe carry out, they can offer their pooches a night on the town at an upscale doggy gourmet deli or restaurant. Here dogs peer at the food in a glass showcase, bark their orders and dine in a booth.

Owners or the dogs choose appetizers, such as guacamole dip with dog biscuit chips, or bite sized pizza shaped treats called Puppizza. They go on to entrees, such as shepherd's pie, steak and kidney ragout or tuna casserole. Then they select side orders such as hush puppies and pupcakes. Finally they decide on dessert, such as chocolate liver chip cookies. Voila ! A four course dinner for Fido! Washed down undoubtedly with bottled water. Unless he insists on fish or beef flavored "Thirsty Dog," a specially formulated pet drink made from purified water and laced with essential vitamins and mineral supplements.

Some frazzled owners won't buy dog food no matter where they find it or how it's packaged because they're overwhelmed by the huge selection. One of my clients said, "I stand in front of the dog food section in the food store feeling like an absolute dummy. I read the labels. I compare ingredients can to can and box to box. How many grams of this and grams of that. Tell me, dammit, what to buy for Clyde!"

Another woman said, "There are too many to choose from. It's easier to cook for Floppy than decide what to buy."

"You have no decision to make," I said. "I'll decide for you." I wrote down a brand and the amount on a slip of paper. She looked at it, and said, "Oh poo! That eliminates the personal touch."

And that's the bottom line.

Feeding a dog is very simple. All it takes is dog food, a bowl, and maybe a can opener. Nothing else. These items, when combined, are enough to make a dog happy. But most doting owners need to add that personal touch because they equate food with love. If they merely open a can and plop the contents into the dog's bowl or their best china and put it on the floor, they're not showing their dog they love him, or that they feel he's important and worthy of time and effort. But put a little or a lot of something in, or heat the food, and soon canine family members are getting more home cooking than the family.

"I get so damned mad at my wife," Saul told me. "She cooks for Pook but not for me."

"Pook appreciates it. You don't," his wife retorted.

"I compliment every damned meal you lower yourself to make for me. I always thank you and tell you it was good."

"If you really meant it, you'd kiss me like Pook does."

Shortly after this, a woman told me, "I get so angry at my husband. He claims he can't boil water to make me a cup of tea but he sautes burgers for the dog, makes him Eggs Benedict and bakes him Spam cookies."

"Hey, you can use the stove," her beloved said. "He can't."

While an occasional people treat is fine for dogs, many owners soon discover than have created a feeding machine. Like the owners of Freida, a Dachshund.

They offered Freida a taste of their bacon and eggs. She licked her chops and begged for more. They gave in. Soon they were making breakfast for three people, not two. Not just any breakfast because Freida would not eat cereals, waffles, pancakes, muffins or bagels. She put in her order every morning for eggs accompanied by bacon, sausage or ham. If she got them she was one happy pup. If she didn't, she showed her displeasure by messing the floor. "Her message is loud and clear," her owners said. After Freida died, a plate of bacon and eggs went into the coffin with her. "It gives us solace to know she went with her favorite foods."

Countless owners cook for their pets, making dog meals from scratch. The efficient chefs prepare enough to freeze several portions. "It's worth it," one client told me. "About half the time she eats what we eat. We eat very simply because of her, things like broiled chicken and rice, or stir-fried veggies with beef, and she likes those. But she won't eat the same meal two nights in a row. So if I plan on having leftovers, all I have to do is open the freezer door and ask Madonna what she wants. Sometimes she doesn't like the first dish I mention but she barks and wags her tail when I come to the meal she wants. I always stock at least three of her favorite entrees. Naturally, she sits at the table with us."

Well, why not? She's just one of many dogs who not only sit at the dinner table but have their own chair.

Ching, a Shih Tzu, was the first "kid" at the table every evening. "He tells us when it's time to eat," I was told. According to his owners, Ching raised his head, shoved his paws over his master's hand and sister's hand and howled before each meal.

"Why's that?" I asked.

"He's saying grace with us."

At least that was one dog who blessed the fact that dog food never passed his lips. Since he preferred meat loaf, broccoli, mashed potatoes and apples, his family ate a lot of meat loaf, broccoli, mashed potatoes and apples. The children begged for macaroni and cheese. They got meat loaf. They asked for carrots. They got broccoli. They got so sick of eating what the dog liked to eat, they moved to Grandma's for two weeks. When they returned, guess what Mom made for them? Meat loaf, broccoli, mashed potatoes and apples.

"How could we possibly change Ching's diet? It would have upset his little tummy."

Not all pampered pets sit on chairs. Some have their own high chair. Others sit on the owner's lap where they're hand fed. Some way out owners go even farther.

A friend who detests dogs called me very early one Monday morning to tell me he had attended a swanky affair. "Leaping Lena," he said, "the dog sat on top of the table! There I was at this fancy dinner party and the hostess puts this dog that looks like a rat on top of a place mat that had a doll saucer on it and while I'm diving into Chateaubriand, so's the rat!"

The dog that joins the family for dinner is usually the dog that wears the bib. "He has to. He's such a little messie," one woman complained while smiling ear to ear. That particular client reserved a red and white checkered bib for the dog's Italian meals, a gold lame bib for dinner parties, and a white lacy job for teatime. Feeling facetious, I said, "I imagine he has matching napkins." He did.

So many owners feel that hairy family members belong at the dinner table they have the rule they all eat together. Occasionally the dog waits for the human dinner hour. More often the family eats when it's the dog's dinner time. What happens if a person isn't home on time? "We eat without my husband. I could never make Mippy wait until daddy gets home."

So, there you have it. All my exceptional clients knew that dog food is the best food for their pets. Most tried their best to adhere to my "dog food and nothing but dog food" rules. Relatively few had success. Even when they barely hung in there I never realized what a challenge it was until the day I overheard two clients talking about feeding their pets.

One was complaining she was a nervous wreck because her old poodle had lost most of his teeth and refused to eat soft dog food when he knew it came out of a can. "If Chip hears the electric can opener, I know we're going to have a fight on our hands."

"You think you have can opener problems?" the second woman said. "My Daphne adores her meals. She hears the electric can opener and gets so excited she hyperventilates and wheezes and triggers off a violent asthma attack."

The first woman ignored the second. "My husband walks Chip so I can open the can, put the food in a pot and warm it. Then when they're back inside, I spoon the food in Chip's bowl. But when the weather's not nice my husband has to entertain him in the bedroom while I use a manual can opener, and I have to make darned sure I don't clank the pot on the stove. It's so hard."

"Hard, my foot. Hard is having a dog that needs a bronchodilator as an appetizer. Hard is having to rush your baby to Dr. Vine so she can get life saving medicine. Hard is sleeping in a bed with a baby who's wheezing from asthma."

"If those dog food makers really cared about animals, they'd have flip off lids on Chip's and Daphne's cans of food. We wouldn't have upset babies every single day."

"We'd be better off, too."

Ironically, that was a week after a hurricane hit town. Each woman mentioned to me in the confines of the examination room that her home had sustained damage. Windows, dishes and breakables in every room had to be replaced. They had done much work to restore order in their homes, and still had not finished. Yet, the sound of the can opener was uppermost on their minds. This is the sign of a real Dog-Gone Owner.

"And I'll never understand them," my friend Gail said. "I think they're made from a different mold than other people."

Gail told me a woman had asked her to poodle sit her "twin girls" for a week. She had accepted, knowing the generous payment she'd receive would help supplement her college income.

Mid-afternoon of day one, the doorbell rang and a delivery boy handed Gail a package. "The owner had instructed me to give each dog two ground sirloin patties, slightly grilled, medium rare. I opened the package and saw four patties. Not five or six. And here I thought I'd be eating sirloin, too."

When she finished cooking, feeding and walking the twins, she looked in the refrigerator for food for herself. "There wasn't any." She looked in the freezer. "It was empty." She looked in the pantry. "I ate canned peas because that's all there was. I foolishly had assumed the owner knew I needed sustenance two or three times a day, but it must have slipped her mind. That night, after walking the twins for the fourth time we went to bed. I had one dog on either side, on their own pillow, breathing hamburger fumes on me. I decided it was every dog for herself.

"The next day the delivery boy handed me four more patties. I went shopping and spent the little cash I had on canned dog food. That night I mixed some with two of the patties, and cooked them for the poodles. They took one smell and walked away. I ate the other two.

"I guess the dogs knew their mistress wasn't there because from the next night on they gobbled up what I gave them, and we both had enough to eat, thanks to the daily delivery. The woman called two or three times to check up on her 'babies.' Not once did she ask what I did for food for the week.

"From then on whenever I dog-sat I gave their owners a price for the service and a food list for me. Believe it or not, more owners never considered my food but spent humongous time telling me what, how and when to feed the dogs. I've baby sat, and take it from me, dog owners are more worried about their pets than people are about their babies. Is that normal?"

Many years later I related Gail's story to a Dog-Gone Owner who looked very confused by the time I reached the end. "I don't understand," he said. What was her problem? That she had to eat peas? I think she was very lucky."

"How's that?" I asked.

"Those pups could have died from eating dog food."

Chapter 3

Steamy Sagas Of Sex

Let's start with a crash course in canine sex. This will help people who are not too knowledgeable about the love life of a dog or the uniqueness of the male dog's genitalia.

First off, it's correct to assume that Fido and Fifi "do it" the way Fred and Freida "do it". But while there are similarities between dog and man, there are also major differences. For example, dogs never assume the missionary position, or any of the dozens of positions humans use for intercourse. They rely totally on the doggy position with the male approaching the female from the rear.

During the normal mating process, the canine's penis enlarges. After the male inserts his penis into the female's vagina, a small bulb on either side of his member swells. These hold the penis snug inside the female during copulation and for 15 to 30 minutes after his climax. When the male calms down, his penis retracts to its normal size and the male and female dogs easily disengage.

Since there's mandatory coupling even after the sex act, the couple cannot immediately separate, roll over on their backs and enjoy a rawhide cigarette. In other words, there is no such thing as a "quickie" in the doggy world.

This fact interested many of my clients who found their dogs philandering with neighborhood sex pots and who called asking me how they could break up these romantic interludes. "I mean, they've been connected forever. Shouldn't I do something?" After I explained dog anatomy, I usually heard them comment, "So that's why they're called 'lucky dogs,' huh?" Occasionally, however, a client had an unusual reaction.

My favorite is the story of Miss Golden, a prim single woman and most difficult client. She let me know in no uncertain terms that she was the medical expert when it came to what was best for her dog, Scarlett. If I said black, she said white. If I said yes, she said no. When I said, "Neuter your dog," she said, "It's totally unnecessary to discuss any form of birth control for Scarlett. She has no use for boys. She's a good girl. Besides," she added, "I don't let her out of my sight when she's 'that way,' " Miss Golden's euphemism for Scarlett's periods of heat.

When Scarlett came into season again, Miss Golden put a pair of her own bloomers on the dog to catch the drops of blood. "I pinned the waist band to make it fit Scarlett." Then, thinking the dog was taking her afternoon nap in her favorite closet, Miss Golden said she made herself a cup of tea. She was standing in front of her breakfast room window, sipping her brew and enjoying the view of her garden when she witnessed a most unexpected sight in the flower bed.

There was Scarlett amid the annuals and perennials, still clad in the bloomers but with a male dog mounted on her back, sharing one of the leg openings and humping her for all he was worth.

I enjoy imagining Miss Scarlett as she dropped her tea cup and broke a track record lunging for the phone to call me. She screamed hysterically, "Scarlett! Scarlett's caught in a trap!"

"What?"

"Trap! Bad boy dog won't let her go!"

She wanted to throw cold water on the dogs to interrupt them. I suggested she bide her time until the dogs separated naturally. Any attempt to dislodge Scarlett from "the trap" could cause painful injuries to both the male and female, I told her. We argued for a few minutes, and in a voice shaking with rage, she said, "I'm looking out the window, Doctor. Separating naturally seems to be taking unnaturally long. But if it will hurt Scarlett to pry that beast out of her, I'll wait." Then before she slammed down the receiver, she sputtered, "That nasty boy should be shot for raping my little girl!"

Despite her trauma, the dog seemed quite content when I saw her a few weeks later. Miss Golden wasn't. "Scarlett and I are now ready to discuss birth control," she informed me.

"And we will," I assured her, "as soon as Scarlett delivers her puppies."

Dogs couldn't care less about choice of mates when they have the urge to copulate. Their only concern is that an easily-aroused male meets a bitch in heat, or vice versa. There's no worry about safe sex, physical appearance, or consideration about choosing a partner of the same breed. Nor is there a commitment to a long term relationship. Leave them alone or give them some slack on their leash and they have little trouble finding mates. This, of course, disturbed many of my Dog-Gone Owners of pedigreed dogs who found that their dogs had mated indiscriminately instead of making the "right" match to produce champion puppies.

The age of modern technology and the computer helped to alleviate that problem when some innovative people created a dating and mating service, a business that boasts it will find the dog of your dreams for your own dog. Owners of studs and bitches anywhere in the United States can register by paying a fee. This allows them to submit their names and phone numbers, and give detailed descriptions of their dog's background and lineage, and special features such as color and size. A representative feeds all information into the computer. Owners interested in selectively breeding their dogs can then purchase a print-out of available mates for their pets and make their choice. One owner contacts the other, and when the bitch is in heat her owner delivers her to the stud. The system works.

Generally, a mating pair does not need assistance. They instinctively know what to do and how to do it. However, every now and then, I had to take an active part in an exceptional patient's love life.

Sir Winston, a massive English bull dog, was in demand by owners of female bull dogs in the United States because he sired fine pups. Unfortunately his large chest and enormous body interfered with his mating. There wasn't a darned thing wrong with his libido, but he had major problems. He couldn't hoist himself up to get into the mating position; he couldn't penetrate the female by himself; he couldn't remain in position long enough to consummate the act; and, he sure as heck couldn't stay put until he became flaccid enough to part from his current flame. That's why two clinic assistants and I had to help Sir Winston with his love life.

After his mistress handed over Sir Winston to me, I'd introduce him to his date of the day, a bitch in heat. While my assistants steadied sexy Winston on top of his eager girl friend, I'd insert his penis so he could do what came naturally. Then the assistants held the dogs together to guarantee their safety until Sir W. was back to his non-sexy self. We repeated the procedure on a regular basis, once or twice a month over several years.

After the first couple of dates, the dog began to associate me with pleasure, a great deal of pleasure, and he refused to perform unless I managed his business end. Familiar with the routine, he was always eager to get the matinee started. He'd take one look at me, tremble from anticipation, jut his chest out even farther, and lead me at a brisk pace into his "boudoir". As soon as I presented him to the female, he'd sniff and grunt a couple of times, and wait for me to do my thing so he could start thrusting. As the finale neared he'd turn his head toward me and lick my face without missing a beat until he climaxed. I don't know if Sir Winston was thanking me or if he had fallen in love with his favorite vet, but I do know it took three people as well as two dogs to start each litter of pups.

Here was a dog that more than earned his keep and loved his job. His mistress was well aware she had one great dog with a talent equalled by few male bull dogs; but being an average owner, she treated his sexuality as nothing out of the ordinary. All he got from her was a pat on the back, a compliment of "What a good boy!" and a ride home so he could take a well-deserved nap. Then both dog and owner forgot about sex until the next stud appointment.

Often, a dog's interest in sex, whether too little, too much or too weird, reared its head and greatly affected worried owners. Consider the sad tale of Murphy, a show dog champion.

Murphy's mistress, Bernice, received numerous offers from dog owners who wanted him to impregnate their females at $1,000 a performance. Many of these eager people had the additional expense of transporting themselves and their bitches to his home town for the affair. The introductions went perfectly, Murphy was cordial and sweet, but he absolutely refused to service the ladies. Time after time Murphy was a dud, completely uninterested and unaroused.

"I don't understand it," Bernice told me. "He's very affectionate, loves to be kissed, wags his tail when I say I love him. He is straight, you know," she said, trying to reassure herself, "he is not gay."

"How do you know?" I asked.

"He often gets sexy with his female stuffed teddy bear. He picks her up and carries her into a corner and tries to have sex with her. He even sleeps with the damn thing. What's wrong with him? He could be as rich as Benji!"

Unfortunately for Bernice, Murphy's love life was complete enough for him. His love for his mistress and his monogamous relationship with his teddy bear precluded amorous encounters with bitches. Bernice became more aggravated after each disastrous date until one day she told me, "I can't take much more of this. Murphy gets one more chance. Either he'll rise to the occasion or he won't."

He didn't. Bernice let him retire with a disappointing track record. "His studding and siring stink," Bernice moaned, "but I still love the little shit."

Nellie was at the other end of the spectrum. Her mistress Marlene started to weep as soon as I entered the examination room. "Look at her," she cried, holding out the poodle. "She's a slut! Bum dogs keep climbing the fence, and she puts out for every one! I'm surprised they didn't stand in line waiting their turn. I have a bordello in my back yard!'' (See illustration 10.)

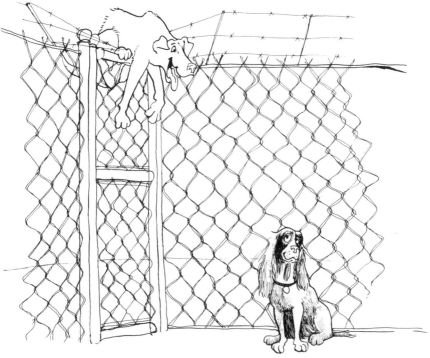

10. Oversexed dog

Instead of fitting Nellie with a chastity belt with a lock and key as Marlene suggested, I ran tests and discovered that ovarian cysts caused the dog's promiscuity. They played havoc with her hormonal system, causing her to come into heat every month or two, and that created her desire to mate. Since Marlene had no plans to breed Nellie, we decided on a hysterectomy to remove her cystic ovaries. Shortly after the surgery Nellie regained her decorum and modesty, and Marlene regained her composure. "Thank God," she said. "Do

you know how embarrassing it was to own the neighborhood trollop?"

I could empathize with Marlene. 99% of dog owners expect
their pet to keep sexual displays behind the "bedroom" door.
It's not nice, they think, to see a dog act like an animal and
impulsively give in to sexual urges.

Yet, much as Dog-Gone Owners profess to know everything about their pets, most don't realize that many dogs face
the same sexual conditions as human beings. Nymphomania,
although not rampant and caused by hormonal disturbance,
does exist in dogdom. Homosexuality is considered ordinary
activity for a lot of puppies until they outgrow adolescence.
Asexuality is another reality although this often goes unno-
ticed until the owners attempt to get the bitch or stud to breed,
like Murphy. Nothing, though, shocks an owner more than
discovering the love of his or her life is changing sex.

Imagine having a Boxer named Elvis and one day noticing
definite changes in his breasts and genitalia. Like Elivis' master, Bernard, you'd probably waste no time calling the vet to
ask, "What the hell is going on?" because, "his nipples aren't
dots anymore, he's got eight gazongas! And his testicles used
to be like hard plums, and now they're like soft olives. And
his bag shrank, it's real wrinkled and tiny. And where the hell
is the hair on his underparts?"

When Bernard brought Elivis in, I didn't know whether to
treat the owner or the dog first. Bernard was so upset about
the changes he was shaking. Why was Elvis, his man dog,
acting like a sissy, squatting "like a girl" when he urinated?
"Tell me Doc, is he gay?" He also mentioned that Elvis
seemed very sad, "like my ex-mother-in-law before we had to
commit her."

From the dog's symptoms I suspected hermaphroditism, a
condition where animals and people possess both male and

female sex organs. Exploratory surgery confirmed my diagnosis. Elvis had functioning ovaries; and thanks to them, he began to produce female hormones until they overtook his normal male hormonal output. No wonder Elvis was confused and depressed. There was only one answer to his problems, and that was to remove his ovaries.

When Bernard picked Elvis up after his surgery, he looked at the dog, sighed, and said, "Let's go home, Elvira."

"Elvira?"

"Well he sure as hell isn't Elvis anymore."

"He still has a penis, though. Why call him Elvira?"

"I don't know what I'm going to call him but I sure as hell am going to call Geraldo Rivera to see if we can get on his show."

When dogs needed help to mate or when their sexual activity was anything out of the ordinary, I was privy to their love lives because of the owners' concerns. The dogs seemed to accept themselves and their sexual orientations, no matter what they were, but it was much harder for their owners. These clients reminded me of overly concerned parents who believed the faults and shortcomings of their children boomeranged back to them and affected their standing in the community. As I often said, I doubted that people outside of their families took the time to psychoanalyze the sexual orientation of their dogs. I never heard one person in Chapel Hill say, "They're the talk of the town. Flibberty is gay because he was the only male sibling in a family of six dogs and his mistress is too domineering." Yet I understood their concerns.

What I could not understand were the invitations I received more times then I cared to count to share the bedrooms of owners. I'm eternally grateful I was never physically there, but I did get verbal blow by blow descriptions of what did or didn't occur there.

The blame for the many National Enquirer revelations always landed on the dogs because they created difficult or impossible situations in the hanky panky department. Consider the case of the missing panties.

A bachelor client who often entertained ladies in his pad called to report, "The damn dog did it again, and my date's really pissed."

"Did what?"

"Stole another pair of her panties. This time, though, he ran off with a bra, too. Every time my date comes here and we end up in the bedroom, the damn dog runs off with her underwear. I just caught him burying her stuff in the back yard."

"Your dog is trying to tell you he's jealous."

"That's his problem," he said. "I'm getting tired of replacing my girl's underwear."

"Try hiding it in a pillowcase or putting it in the closet," I suggested.

"Tried both. Didn't work."

"Throw the damn things on a high shelf."

"Thanks, doctor, I'll try it," he said, "if I remember."

He must have solved his problem because he didn't call back for more suggestions.

Not all couples, however, could solve their bedroom doggy problems as easily. Depending on the disposition of the dogs, it could take a long time to find a solution that was acceptable to both man and beast. This was the situation with Dan, who after his divorce got custody of Angus. Each time Dan brought a woman home, his jealous dog growled and tried to bite her. Dan didn't object much until he fell in love with Lucy and wanted to marry her. Then the dog's obvious dislike of the woman presented quite a problem.

Dan and Lucy came in for a consultation. We decided to try a little behavior modification. I suggested that Lucy try a lot of TLC, tender love and care. She was to feed Angus, and try to pet him. That helped some, but not enough.

"It's a shame your ex didn't leave any of her clothes in the house," I casually mentioned to Dan one day when he called.

"She left a few things," he answered.

"Anything that she might have worn but not washed?"

"A ratty looking pair of shorts. Maybe a T-shirt or two."

"Do you think Lucy would be willing to wear some of them so Angus picks up the scent of your ex?"

Lucy wasn't overjoyed at the idea, but she agreed to try it. The day came when both the TLC and the clothes worked, and Angus mellowed a bit. Gradually he changed his opinion of Lucy and eventually he grew to love her. At last report, they were still compatible.

Other dogs, however, refused to come around. Overly possessive and jealous of their special person, they were responsible not only for the high percentage of couples who slept in separate beds but also for giving the kiss of death to quite a few marriages or relationships.

Sparky, a Cairn Terrier, for example, hated Joe as much as he adored Joe's wife, Mina. Whenever the couple hugged or kissed, Sparky wedged himself between them. Mina thought it was funny that Sparky jumped in bed with her and growled at Joe. "He dares me to jump under the sheets," Joe said. "It isn't worth it. I sleep in the guest bedroom." (See illustration 11)

But on one wedding anniversary Joe told Sparky, "I don't care what the hell you do; I'm sleeping with my wife in my bed." Sparky, not accustomed to hearing Joe raise his voice, woofed softly, but allowed Joe to get into bed. Mina reported the couple progressed very slowly "to give Sparky time to

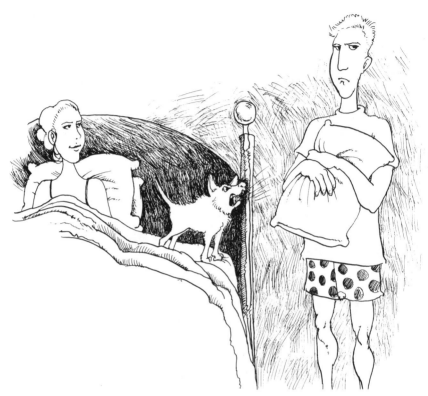

11. Dog barking at husband approaching bed

adjust." But when Joe was beginning to enjoy himself and had forgotten about the dog in his bed, Sparky lifted a leg and urinated on him. That was it for Joe, who soon found solace with a lady who was allergic to dogs. (See illustration 12.)

Because Dog-Gone Owners feel their pets are people, too, many insist this entitles their dogs to share the marital bed each night. If the significant others were equally tolerant or

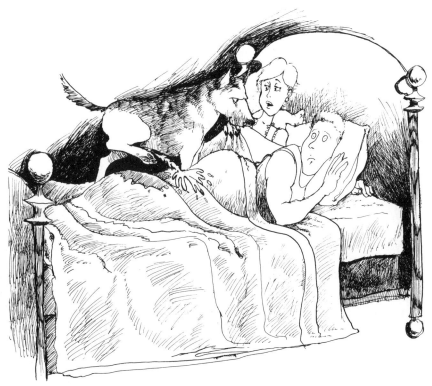

12. Jealousy rears its ugly head

loved the dogs, the transition from two to three or more in the same bed posed no problem. But some considered the togetherness a treat for special occasions.

Mitzi Lou's mistress and master, for example, didn't regard the poodle as a nuisance. Yet, she slept in a miniature version of their brass bed, except when the couple wanted to make love. Then Bobby Joe would tell Mitzi Lou "to get on his pillow."

Understanding her signal, she'd make herself comfortable on Bobby Joe's pillow. Then she'd extend one paw for Ruth

Lee, her mistress, to hold during intercourse and squeeze at the moment of orgasm. To Ruth Lee this was the epitome of bliss, to be intimate and in physical contact with the two "people" she loved most in the world. Maybe this arrangement was unorthodox, but it was harmonious and pleasurable for all three.

At times, though, sleeping with an animal or animals can put a damper on a couple's love life as Betty and Barney discovered.

For years they slept with two large dogs in a double bed and insisted it did not restrict their love life. The last time they told me this, I decided to confront the chubby couple.

"It has to restrict you a little bit," I argued, "because those dogs are big."

"Nope, not at all. They both stay as still as they possibly can. They're very considerate."

Shortly after this talk their male German Shepherd, Bogart, had a stroke and became partially paralyzed in his back legs. As his nerve disintegration increased, the dog began to dribble more and more urine. As if this wasn't bad enough, their female German Shepherd, Blossom, became incontinent because of old age, and she, too, began to leak like a faucet.

Then Betty began to complain. She and Barney hadn't been able to make love since the dogs lost bladder control. "They seem to have perfect timing," she said. "The second Barney and I get in the mood, we're flooded out of bed."

"Why don't you move to another bed?" I asked.

"You've got to be kidding!" she said, "our babies have slept with us every night since we brought them home."

"Then put diapers on them."

"No way," Betty said, "that would hurt their feelings. They're embarrassed enough now."

"It can't be much fun trying to make love in a wet bed."

"It isn't. We're constantly interrupted. Besides that, we have to get up several times each night to strip the bed, change linens and do laundry."

They finally agreed they had to do something. "No diapers, though." They resolved the problem to some degree by pinning absorbent Turkish towels around the dogs. "Damp isn't so bad," Barney told me, showing me the tolerance and generosity of an unconventional owner.

Many significant others, however, not having been put to the test and being madly in love, thought they'd easily jump over any canine hurdle that stood in their way. All they had to do was thaw out a jealous pet that resented sharing a mistress or master and mattress, and prove to the person that human love and companionship beat a dog's any day.

What the newcomer to the "menage a trois " didn't understand was that the owner and pet had gotten along just fine before the "outsider" arrived. The one expected to adjust was the newcomer who parked shoes under the unfamiliar bed, not the mistress or the master, or the dog.

Often Dog-Gone Owners tried to clarify this from the start. Before they committed to a relationship with one special human being, they insisted on a pre-nuptial or pre-cohabitation agreement. I saw a few. The wording of the agreement varied, but the content didn't. They all meant, "If you love me, you'll love my pet no matter what and don't you ever forget it."

Anna insisted her fiancee sign a pre-nuptial agreement concerning her pets. Larry didn't object that Anna's pony could come into the house whenever he pleased. At least the contract stipulated he was to sleep in the stable. Larry even agreed that the dwarf donkey could sleep in the bedroom. At least it stipulated that he was to sleep in a large dog bed. What ticked him off was item number three. Larry was to share the bed with his wife and her seven dogs.

Fed up with a crowded bed and inhaling dog hair through 10 years of marriage, Larry finally rebelled. "It's them or me!" he insisted. Anna chose her pets over her husband and merely said, "Good riddance! He snored too loud, anyway."

The attitude that a dog was the same or better than any man . . . or woman . . . was and is common among extreme owners. Many of these clients fell into my "humdinger" category because I saw absolutely no difference in sexual behavior between them and their dogs.

Here I speak mainly of men. While my female clients worried about their dogs' unusual sexual orientation such as being gay or oversexed, I rarely heard them complain about a male or female dog's celibacy. Interestingly, male clients believed in a double standard. Their female dogs could remain virginal through life without missing anything, but their male dogs needed sex. Just as what was good for the goose was good for the gander, the prevalent belief was that what was good for the male owner was good for the male dog. Aware of it or not, the men attributed their own attitudes, beliefs and appetites to their male dogs.

A good example of this is Mr. Schwartz, a gentleman in his early 70s. Mr. Schwartz repeatedly vetoed the suggestion to alter his Doberman although castration is a standard procedure when owners don't want their male dogs to urinate on furniture, wander away from home or impregnate bitches. "You can't de-ball Gismo! You'll take away his manhood!"

Mrs. Schwartz called me one day to say her husband had changed his mind. "Listen," she told me, "I told Sidney that if Gismo has the operation he won't squat like a sissy when he makes a wee-wee. Am I right? He'll still lift a leg?"

"You're right, he'll still act like a male."

Mrs. Schwartz relayed the news to Mr. Schwartz who got on the phone, and said, "Then, cut off his balls, dammit."

Post surgery, Gismo became depressed and Mr. Schwartz became more depressed. Mrs. Schwartz brought both of her guys in to see me.

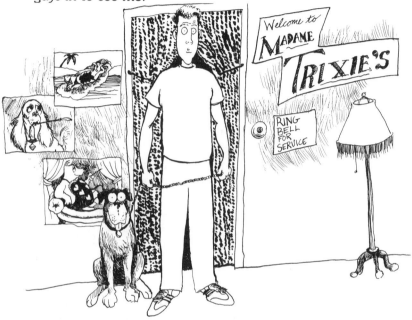

13. Cat house for dogs

"I understand why Gismo's sad," she said. "He knows something's missing, he has a right to be depressed. But him?" she said, pointing to her husband, "He still has his. They work. Maybe not as good as they did 50 years ago, but what's the big deal?"

"I told you a thousand times I can't enjoy using mine when Gismo doesn't have any to use," Mr. Schwartz said. "It's a macho thing. Gismo's is suffering because he doesn't have the balls to prove he's a male. That poor guy!"

My advice to the couple was to surgically insert a pair of silicon prosthetic testicles called neuticals into Gismo's scrotum to make him appear like a normal male. Mrs. Schwartz threw her hands up in the air and said she thought the idea of subjecting the dog to surgery again was unnecessary and ridiculous. "Gismo's lost his ammunition, understand? Silicon won't give him back live cannon balls or hormones."

Mr. Schwartz prevailed, and his wife gave in. "I think it's crazy," she told him, "but it's worth it if it will put a smile back on your face."

Gismo's surgery restored Mr. Schwartz' smile. The prostheses helped the Doberman and the husband recover, and they resumed their walks through the neighborhood struttin' their stuff. "He's got all the other dogs fooled, Doc." That ended Mr. Schwartz's preoccupation with his pet's sex life.

Not so with other male clients who felt they had to guarantee an active and regular sex life for their male dogs, even when females weren't in the vicinity.

Mr. Anonymous confided to me that he allowed his male dog to hump his leg once a week until the dog had an orgasm because "he needs the sexual release, Doc." I didn't ask if he conferred with the dog or not beforehand, but I suspect it was the owner's idea.

Mr. I'll Nevertell divulged that because he believed in safe sex he donned rubber gloves before he masturbated his dog once a week. He scheduled the event for Sunday evenings believing "he should start out the week nice and relaxed." Again, the dog wasn't consulted. But it was the macho thing for a macho dog.

What this points out to me is that in the area of sex some bizarre owners will do anything to give their pets the same pleasures they relish. If you're wondering if any owners went as far as to include intercourse or oral sex with their pets, the answer is yes. The dogs were taught to satisfy their favorite person's sexual desires. Surprising as that might be, it surprised me more that clients told me about it.

As far back as the 1950s I had read Dr. Kinsey's report that four percent of dog owners acknowledged indulging in some form of sexual practice with their pets. If four percent admitted it, I suspect the actual percentage was more then, and probably higher today. Somehow I can't see everyone who fooled around with their pets, once or frequently, raising their hands and yelling, "Count me in, too!" I'm sure there are people out there who consider their sex lives private, especially when it involves an animal. No matter what the numbers are, however, I presume they reflect the owners' benefits rather than the dogs'.

It's undeniable that some owners also get vicarious thrills through their dogs. That explains the success of a business like a Greenwich Village establishment, a "cathouse" for dogs. One client told me he had taken his dog there several times while he lived in New York. (See illustration 13.)

The name describes exactly what it is. For $100.00 the proprietor, Joe Scaggs, provided a male dog with a female companion that was in a state of artificially induced heat. When the dogs went into action, the resident photographer did, too, unless the owner brought his camera. Either way, dog owners had permanent mementos of the occasion.

Mr. Scaggs guaranteed complete satisfaction. If the male dog couldn't perform in the "cat house," he brought a female to the male's turf where he felt more comfortable.

Why on earth would anyone open a business like this? Mr. Scaggs believed he filled a need in the canine community. I believe he also realized there were enough kinky dog owners to take advantage of his service.

He's not the only person to cater to a specialized clientele; consider the magazines that concentrate on bestial pornography. Creative people in this field blatantly announce they fill a need in the human community by giving unconventional folks what they want.

In time I thought I had heard everything. Then Luigi became my patient and other clients practices seemed tame in comparison to his mistress.

Priscilla was a single woman in her 40s. Outwardly she seemed like a typical owner, very concerned with her young Pomeranian. Then, during Luigi's examinations, she began to startle me with unusual comments, such as, "He's really well hung, isn't he, Doc?"

Let's be realistic. A Pomeranian will never be able to compete with a German Shepherd or Mastiff, but I guess size is in the eyes of the beholder.

Another time, she described in detail Luigi's fondness for masturbation. He enjoyed doing it in front of people, she said. He also loved to mount anything that moved or didn't move. "Do you encourage him?" I asked.

"Well it is funny as all get out," she admitted.

"You should stop encouraging him," I admonished.

When Luigi was about four or five years old, she said, "Doc, you have to see him in action when I have parties."

She explained how she had trained Luigi to entertain her guests. She'd tell him "go get kitty." Hearing the command, he'd run and proudly bring back a stuffed cat that he used as a sexual partner until he reached a climax and ejaculated. "My guests love the side show. They laugh and applaud. Of course there are always are few party poopers who tell me they're disgusted or horrified."

Having a client like Priscilla made me appreciate all the more those adoring owners who went out of their way to shield their dogs. One was Mrs. Zeller, a woman in her late 60s, who felt it was immoral for her Snookums to witness the sex act. Therefore, before she and her husband enjoyed an interlude of intimacy, Hubby took Snookums for a long walk to tire the dog and ensure he'd fall into a deep sleep and snore loud enough to block out any love sounds.

"It works like a charm," said Mrs. Zeller, "even though the exercise is so strenuous to Hubby these days he needs a little time to recuperate before he has the energy to perform."

Then there was Mrs. Tillman who spelled out "nervous" words, like s-o-r-e (as in nipple) or c-l-o-g-g-e-d (as in anal glands). A third considerate person was Donna Worth who insisted we sing our way through all of Bonnie's pre-natal appointments. "It has to be to the tune of 'Mary Had A Little Lamb' because that's her favorite and keeps her calm." But, the corker of all was Rose Drucker who brought in her Pug, Daisy.

"She's getting married in the morning," said Mrs. Drucker.

"Oh, I didn't know she was engaged. Congratulations, Daisy!" I answered.

"She's a little nervous, Dr. Vine. I brought her in so you can assure me she's up to it."

"Are you talking about the mating?"

"Well, Daisy's a virgin, she has never even seen a male's whatzitz, let alone made love."

"Hum," I said, nodding my head. I examined Daisy and told Mrs. Drucker, "She's in fine shape. You have nothing to worry about."

"That's good to hear, but I've got to ask you one more thing. Is it true that Daisy and her husband will remain joined for 15 to 30 minutes after he consummates the act?"

"It's true."

"Well," she said, leashing Daisy's collar, "thank you for reassuring me."

"You're welcome."

"Fifteen to 30 minutes," she mumbled on her way out. "Fifteen to 30 whole minutes. Daisy, no wonder they call dogs lucky!"

Chapter 4

Glitz and Glamour

As a veterinarian I never suggested that dog owners dress their pets. I believe a natural fur coat plus the demure accessory of a small identification tag attached to a neutral leather or woven collar is appropriate for any formal or informal occasion. Certainly it was appropriate for bringing the dog to my clinic for treatment or a checkup.

Considering the impact that clothing designers have had on fashion- minded men and women since Eve paved the way in the Garden of Eden, it was logical that some of my Dog-Gone Owners would dress their dogs as well if not better than they dressed themselves.

I never paid much attention to the attire of my patients until I had occasion to see Sadie, a very healthy terrier. By the fifth visit I noticed that every time I saw Sadie she wore a different collar while her mistress held a matching leash. Some things become harder to ignore, so I finally commented on the collars.

"I've seen five. Does she have seven? One for each day of the week?"

"Well, no," said her mistress. "She only has five, one for each of her moods."

"Oh?" I said.

"Yes. When she's happy, she wears pink. When she's depressed, she wears blue. When she's excited, she wears the red set. When she's jealous of our grandson, she wears the green."

"What about this one with the blue and red stripes?"

"She's going through menopause, like me. We're both nervous wrecks today. It's funny," she said with a puzzled look on her face, "how our good days and our bad days always coincide."

"Um hum," I commented as I started to clip Sadie's nails. "Does she wear different collars the same day?"

"Oh yes, she's very moody. I have to watch her carefully."

The thought occurred to me that I could send Sadie a birthday present, a jazzy number with multi-colored zigzags to celebrate her future schizophrenia, but I thought better of it.

While Sadie had her collars and leashes, some of my other patients had the basic weather wardrobe. Nothing fancy. A few sported "Who's a bitch?" and "Call me stud" T-shirts on beautiful spring and autumn days. More wore a light-weight fabric poncho on windy days, a water repellant coat on rainy days, and a sweater or two on nippy days. One fashion plate, though, wore his winter snowsuit and boots for the three-minute car trip from his indoor garage to my clinic. "You can never be too careful," Clarence's mistress told me as she unzipped his hood.

Judging from the thousands of photographs of dogs I admired over the years, a lot of time, care and money was invested into the dogs' clothing. It wasn't enough for some Dog-Gone Owners to outfit their pets according to weather conditions. They also dressed them for social occasions and holidays. Dressing the dogs must have been great fun for owners who wanted lasting memories of their pets dressed to the hilt and posed next to the prop of the day. So out came the cameras.

One questionable photographic star was Buster Rottweiler. There he was on a heart shaped rug, wearing a heart shaped hat and coat, with a heart shaped "I Love U" sign hanging on his chest. Flip the page, and there was Buster in his Easter coat and bonnet. Turn more pages and there he was in his Mother's Days cape, his Father's Day crown and his Fourth of July Flag costume. By the time I reached Christmas with Buster in his Santa Claus outfit, and New Years Eve with Buster in a top hat and bow tie, I was sure Buster had hoped for something stronger than water to celebrate the coming year.

Clearly, Buster's "Mommy" didn't agree. When I returned the album to her, she held it to her breast and crooned, "Isn't he adorable? He's my little ham. He just loves it when he sees me coming with the camera."

Kidding on the square, I told her, "One of these days he's going to get you!" Then I tried to forget I had ever seen Buster dressed anyway but au natural.

Several months later I received a phone call from Buster's Mommy who was sobbing so uncontrollably she could not talk. While I waited for her to pull herself together I mentally wrote a tragic scenario. Buster was dead. He had come to an abrupt and horrifying end. He had dashed out into traffic. He had tried to eat an electric cord. Maybe he had swallowed the contents of the freezer without thawing out the food. "Please," I begged her, "tell me what happened."

"He piddled!" she exploded. "He piddled in the box where I keep all his beautiful outfits!"

"A little or a lot?"

"A little? Have you ever seen a Rottweiler pee a little? It was like Niagara Falls!" she said. "He looked me straight in the eye, lifted a leg, aimed, and let go right in front of me!"

As the saying goes, "What goes around, comes around" and it's usually deserved.

Many owners considered dog attire a necessity, not an option, and the dog's clothing allowance was considered part of the family's clothing budget. That, of course, determined the extent and quality of the dogs' wardrobe. Some owners claimed their dogs didn't seem to mind if they had to wear hand-me-downs or even go without fashionable duds, but others maintained their classy pups complained if they weren't outfitted in a new creation or the latest design.

"Snooks is a snob," his mistress told me. "He loves his raincoat and his rain hat, and now that he's used to his rubber booties he insists on wearing them. But you know, he still doesn't like to go outside in the rain even though I hold an umbrella over him."

"Oh?" I commented, "I can't imagine why."

"I know why," she said, looking most annoyed. "He's angry because I won't buy him a new raincoat with a matching or color coordinated attached umbrella. Those stupid designers should be killed!"

"Hum," I replied.

When it came to discussions about doggy haute couture I relied heavily on "Oh," and "Hum." They seemed fairly safe as far as responses go, and could be interpreted any way the owner wanted. But there was one time I ventured beyond monosyllables.

Herman, a 110 pound German Shepherd, was brought to me for a check-up in January. "The Missus and I don't know what's wrong with him," said his master, "but look at him." I looked. Herman stood in front of me with his head bowed and his tail between his legs.

"Hum," I said, nodding my head.

"He used to be a real dog," his owner continued. "He couldn't wait to go outside and attack every dog in the neighborhood. I mean, he'd see those dogs through the living room window and he'd growl and look as if he wanted to rip their throats out. You know what I mean?" I nodded again.

"And now I have a hard time getting him outside to do his business. You know what I mean? I gotta drag the damn dog outside. Really drag him outside." Then he voiced his concern in a whisper so Buster couldn't hear. "He's gonna get a bladder or kidney infection," he hissed. "Know what I mean? He could get impacted, too. Know what I mean?" I decided to keep on nodding to let the gentleman know I really knew what he meant.

After examining Herman, I started to write up the report, and said, "There's nothing physically wrong with him, but he does look and act depressed. Is anything wrong at home? Did something happen that upset him? Is your wife away? Can you tell me anything?"

"Nope, Doc. Not a damn thing. You know what I mean?"

I suggested he bring Herman back the following week so we could see what was what. As I continued to write my notes, the gentleman took his coat off a hanger and put it on. I patted Herman goodbye and turned to shake the man's hand. Then I noticed he was holding something.

"What's that?" I asked.

"That's Herman's custom-made fur coat," the gentleman said, holding it out for me to admire. "Isn't it a beauty? It cost a bundle. Know what I mean?"

I reached for the coat and held it under Herman's nose. "Do you like this coat, Herman?" The dog moaned, backed up as far as he could go, and looked positively miserable.

I invited the gentleman to sit down for a little conference, and laid into him unmercifully. "Herman does not need a fur coat, off the rack or custom-made." I told him. "He already has one."

He nodded.

"How would you like to wear two fur coats? Oh, you wouldn't? Well, that's what you're making your dog do. Now all the other dogs think he's a sissy. You've emasculated him by making him wear this. If you really love your dog, you'll donate this to Salvation Doggy. Know what I mean?"

He knew. He handed me the coat and said, "Ditch it."

The minute I threw it out of the room, Herman's head and tail stood at attention. He wagged his hind quarters and literally pranced out of the room. He was 110 pounds of proud masculinity again.

I've yet to hear of dogs carrying a canine fashion magazine to their owners and indicating via a pointed paw or tail that they were dying to wear a particular number. But I've heard many owners report that their dogs were out of sorts until they were dressed as people.

Fifi adored socializing if she could show off her diamond collar and sequined jump suit. But if she only had a fancy bow around her neck and nail polish on her nails Fifi felt half-dressed, said her owner, adding that she refused to poke her head out of the wicker basket that her mommy used as a doggy seat. Bibzee's owner claimed her dog pouted unless she received a new hair ribbon every week. And Florrie went on hunger strikes if her mistress bought an article of clothing for herself but nothing for her dog. "She was telling me I can't expect her to wear old rags when I don't." Needless to say, these owners quickly learned to dress their dogs and dress them well.

In each case, the owners dictated the dogs' dress codes. Designer dogs were interesting and often comical to see, especially if they and their owners enjoyed being the center of attention. Sometimes, in the case of a shy owner, it was easier to break the ice with strangers when they brought an easygoing and well-dressed pet to a social setting.

These men, usually unmarried young men in their 20s and 30s, routinely dressed their pets in sun glasses, a bandana and a hat for a game of Frisbee on the beach. "It catches the eye of lots of nice looking women," was the reason they gave. One man claimed all he had to do to attract the opposite sex was stick a specially made backpack on his dog and go on a hike. "It worked every time," he claimed. (See illustration 14.)

Maybe that accounts for the bachelors, but quite a few of the married men went further. One client, Terrence, told me he went horseback riding accompanied by his collie. But Rusty would not mount his custom made saddle atop a horse until his custom made derby was plunked on his head. "It didn't take me long to catch on," said Terrence.

Pookie, a Yorkie, wouldn't raise a paw when a golf ball whizzed by unless he was wearing his "fore" cap. The cap made him feel like a real golfer said his owner and that's all he needed to chase a ball down the fairway. His master also said Pookie wouldn't get into the Jacuzzi unless he was wearing his custom-made life jacket. That clever dog, he told me, was frightened by water but realized the life jacket enabled him to float. (See illustration 15.)

One owner holds my record for going all the way.

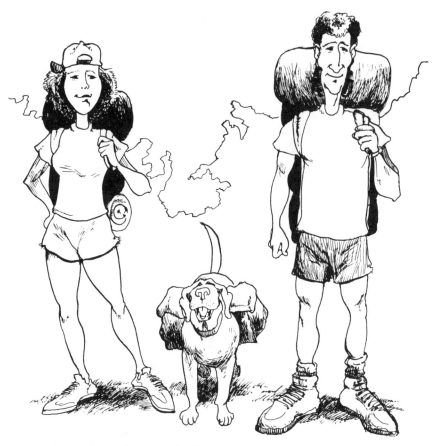

14. Back-packing with dog

From the moment Chuck and Pal saw each other in a shelter they knew they were meant for each other. "I never felt this strong surge of love when I met a woman, but it was there when I saw this mongrel looking at me and wagging his tail." To this day Chuck will tell you that "Pal isn't just one of my friends; he is my best friend. We do everything together."

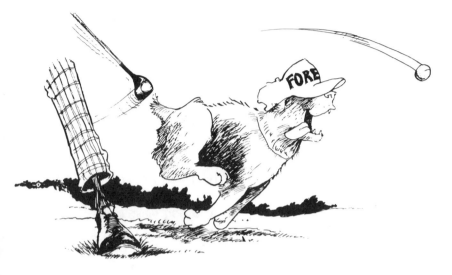

15. Golfing dog

In order to do everything together, Pal had to be as well dressed and protected as his master. So during car rides the dog wore goggles and a long scarf that billowed in the wind, and sat in a specially constructed seat that allowed him to stick his nose out the sun roof.

When Pal went skiing with his owner he wore his goggles and a specially tailored zippered jacket for his sweeps down snow trails. His feet were snugly protected in child-sized sneakers on his custom made 42" skis.

During the summers when it was time to enjoy water sports, Chuck packed two duffel bags, one for himself and the second for Pal's attire and equipment. "Well, Pal needs bathing suits and his towels, sunglasses and his custom made life jacket for speed boat rides," Chuck said. And goggles replaced the sunglasses before Pal stepped on his custom made water skis.

"If we go scuba diving, he wears his special rubber jacket and an oxygen tank that feeds air through to a plastic see-through bubble that keeps his head dry. Believe it or not, he's at my side on the floor of the ocean, walking around, investigating the sea life, and having the time of his life."

When I asked how he managed to convince Pal to dress for each sport, Chuck insisted it was the dog's idea. "He'd bring my stuff over to me, and when I'd get dressed he'd sort of growl under his breath. So one day I put a hat on his head and a scarf around his neck, and he kissed me. I'd say he told me, wouldn't you?"

All right, so maybe dressing up a dog wasn't always the owner's idea.

The more I heard and saw the more I thought it was unnecessary to humanize canines. But there is always an exception to every rule. I speak specifically of "doggie britches."

Doggie britches are for the female dog that is in heat. They weren't much to look at when they first became available. The most important features were that they made the dog "male proof" and that an owner could tuck a facial tissue inside to absorb the small amount of blood the female discharged.

Today, they're fashion items, thanks to the designers. While they still serve the same purposes, a Dog-Gone Owner can lose her mind trying to find the ideal pair for her dog. "It's more confusing than trying to decide on one box of cereal or one can of soup," a client told me.

I've seen women stand in front of the display and heard them talk out loud to themselves as they've tried to narrow down their decisions. Don't quote me, as the following monologue isn't verbatim, but it's close enough to prove my point.

"Well, let's see, Fong Che Non is definitely a mid-sized Char Pei. She probably wears a medium size. Solid or patterned? Solid. Goes with more accessories. Would she like white? No, gets dirty too soon, and she's such an immaculate girl. Yellow? Ugh, she hates yellow. Blue? Looks nice on her but people might think she's a boy. It's hard to tell with Char Peis. OK, I'll get pink. Oh look, they have the pink with ruffles! And, pink with lace! Which should I buy? The ruffles will accentuate her bottom. She doesn't need that. Oh shoot. Do they have the pink in the bikini cut with lace? Hope so, because she does have cute legs. Won't hurt to show them off. Yes, here they are! I'll have her initials monogrammed on them. Or shouldn't I? Maybe that will call more attention to her having her period. So what? She's a woman."

By the time an owner finally connects Fong Che Non to her panties they will definitely be a fashion item.

As the years rolled by, I slowly began to accept dressed-up dogs. While I never changed my belief that they were not people and, therefore, didn't need to be dressed in people clothes, I heard myself defending these pets and their owners. It made sense, sometimes darned good sense, if it was done for a better reason than status.

Consider, for example, Hortense O'Rourke. Hortie was an unmarried, childless woman who treated her dog like a baby. Every day she dressed Clementine in layette clothes, propped her on pillows in a baby buggy, tucked a blanket around her, and wheeled her to the park for her constitutional.

Clementine was relaxed, looked comfortable and, judging from the tail that wagged under the blanket, plainly enjoyed being Hortense's baby. The other half of the "odd couple" had a reason to get up, get dressed and get out every morning. Through her dressed up baby and her walks she avoided the loneliness and isolation that is so common among octogenarians. Clementine was Hortie's reason to keep going. She was a 24 hour a day project. And, she also benefitted the community as she brought smiles to more than one sourpuss who stopped to talk to her.

Another exception to the no-dress rule was a happily married couple in their retirement years, Bill and Margaret Thompson. Their one sadness was that they were not able to have children. Instead, they adopted four dogs: Susie, Patricia, Henry and Frankie.

Bill and Margaret dressed their "kids" in children's clothes that had been altered to fit. Inside their house, the "girls" wore skirts and blouses or dresses, and the "boys" were pants and shirts. They all wore pajamas to bed. Outside, each dog wore his or her own hat, raincoat or fur-lined coat, and rubber boots. These dogs were their babies, as real to them as any sons and daughters could be. They were inseparable, spoke baby talk to them, served them people food at the table, made sure they had a doggy education, and even put money aside for their futures.

Two people created their family dream, and four dogs found loving "parents." While this isn't an unusual occurrence between Dog-Gone Owners and their dogs, what set the Thompsons apart from most others was the mutual respect and great affection that continually flowed between the human beings and the dogs. This love affair benefited all concerned.

Somehow it didn't seem at all strange when you saw Margaret straighten Susie's outfit so her tail could poke out of her skirt, or Bill motion Frankie over so he could adjust the suspender that had slipped off his shoulder.

Dressing dogs is nothing new. You'll always see it. But, I'm afraid you might see more radical styles as fashion designers have their way and owners run to buy the latest fads.

According to a recent fashion show for the woman who has everything, a new trend is to coordinate human and canine attire. One guest in the audience reported that an unforgettable couple in the show had enough polka-dots to send her running to the eye doctor for a checkup. The model's dress, hair ribbon, shoes and handbag were red with black polka dots. The dog's hair ribbon, collar and leash matched her outfit. I thought it was funny until I heard that the white poodle's hair had been dyed red with black polka-dots painted on.

The problem with this for those who can afford it is that too many people are carried away by the look without realizing that it's potentially harmful to the dog.

A few days after I heard about this fashion spectacular, a client came to the clinic with her magnificent standard poodle, Alberta. Alberta had a standing Friday morning appointment for a manicure with my groomer who was next door, and usually dropped by with her owner to say hello.

I could see that Alberta's nails had as usual been filed to perfection and were painted to coordinate with the collar and accessories she'd wear in the coming week. Sometimes she padded in with red or pink polish. Other times it was green, black, or blue. Occasionally her nails were painted in metallics, with or without sparkles, stones, or decorative tape. This day, though, I noticed that her nails were gold with silver accents. They matched her owner's.

"Aha!" I said. "You two must have a special social event to attend."

"Right! We're going to my brother's wedding in New York."

"She's a beautiful dog," I told her, "with or without nail polish."

"Oh, I know she is. Can you see it?"

"See what?"

"Alberta broke a nail. Darn, right before the wedding, too. But Lynn put on a fake claw nail. Can you notice?" When I shook my head, she said, "Good." Then she continued, "I just got a great idea. It will have to wait until we return home but I want you to dye Alberta's hair pink to match my Cadillac."

"What?!"

"Dye her fur pink. And, I want my initials clipped into her fur."

"Did you by any chance attend a fashion show recently?"

"Yes."

"Was there a white poodle that had been dyed red? Black polka dots painted on?"

"How did you know?" she asked.

"Don't worry about that, but worry about the effects of the hair dye on Rene." I explained the good chance of the dog developing hives or a rash that itched like crazy. "Is it worth it just to have a pink poodle?"

There's no doubt that adorning a dog is usually harmless when the adornment is confined to clothing and the dog likes the idea. It does elevate the owner's esteem because a dressed up dog commands a lot of attention, be it a smile, chuckle or occasional gasp. But as in all things, there is a time and place for it.

For example, I don't believe that it's necessary for a dog to announce his religion by wearing an embroidered yarmulke (skull cap) to signify he's Jewish, or a hat embellished with a cross to signify that she's Catholic or Protestant. But if you do, and if that dog shares your dinner table for the Sabbath or a religious holiday, please make sure the hat is securely but not too tightly fastened around your pet's head with an elastic strap. The last thing you need is a hat falling in with the matzo balls or noodles in the soup bowl. That could ruin the spirituality and start the hilarity.

You know what I mean?

Chapter 5

Hooked On The Habit

Right now anyone who is addicted to a drug of choice can attend a self-help group. Among them:

Alcoholics Anonymous (AA), Overeaters Anonymous (OA), Gamblers Anonymous (GA), Narcotics Anonymous (NA), Sex Addicts Anonymous (SA), and Chocoholics Anonymous (CA).

Now here's a new one for you—Anonymous Dogs Under The Influence, or A-DUTI.

Perhaps I'm exaggerating the point a little, but it makes sense that a group such as this is in our future, say around 2000 AD, when many Dog-Gone Owners and members of AA, OA, NA, SA and CA will have inadvertently or deliberately hooked their pets on their same drugs of choice. The only folks who don't have to worry about passing on their "habit" are Gamblers Anonymous as dogs have no end of trouble shuffling and dealing cards, throwing dice and guessing odds.

The large number of addicted dogs has already given rise to a distinctive group of "sick" jokes:

How do you know if your dog likes marijuana? Blow the smoke in her face. If she turns her nose up and walks away, she's clean. If she sniffs it, licks her lips and drools, she wants a joint.

How do you know if your dog is a compulsive overeater? If he eats his dinner, then studies every morsel of food going into your mouth with intense longing, chews his way through a closed storage container to get to 20 pounds of loose kibble, eats until he throws up and then begs for more food, he's a foodaholic.

How do you know if your dog is a hung-over alcoholic? If he's listless, bleary eyed, appears to have a headache, covers his head with his paws and moans as he breathes, BUT perks up when you offer him another drink, or as I like to call that, "a hair of the dog," he's a drunk. (See illustration 16.)

Finally, how do you know if your dog is a pill head? If she raids the medicine cabinet and swallows only those containers holding uppers, downers or painkillers, she's a substance abuser.

Joking aside, an increasing number of dogs are addicted to one thing or another. Sometimes inconsiderate owners give their dogs "uppers" or "downers" when they themselves indulge. (See illustration 17). Other times the cause is heredity. For example, some breeds of dogs seem to be born chow hounds or compulsive overeaters. They can't get enough even when they've had too much. But when you add environment (people) to heredity, you can end up with a dog whose mouth never shuts.

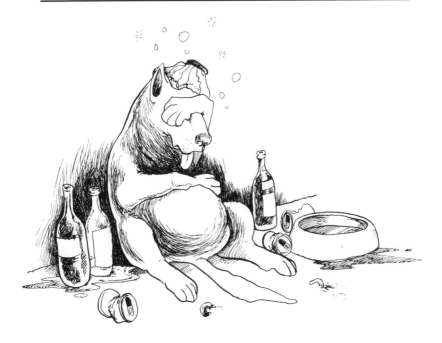

16. A sneaky party drinker

Gomer Sue Beagle is a textbook example of a compulsive overeater. Had her owners not emphasized food, Gomer still would have gone crazy when she saw her mistress dishing out her meals. She still would have have gulped down her dinner in 90 seconds and let everyone know it was the highlight of her day. And she still would have begged for more food, too.

As it was, Gomer's owners were a young couple who treated her like a baby to the point where they carried her infant style with her head on their shoulders or cuddled her belly up in their arms. Then the couple had a real baby. To make sure Gomer didn't feel jealous, they began to give her

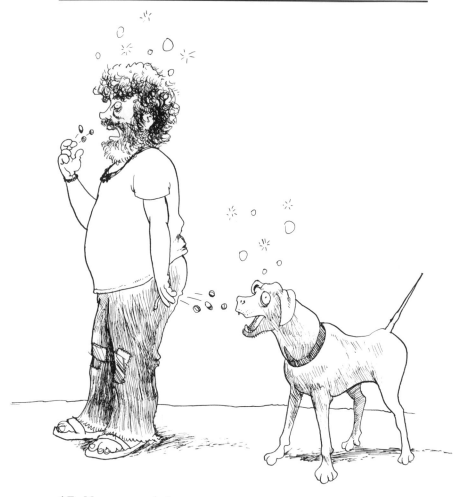

17. Uppers and downers

a treat every time they fed their child or themselves. "Just a little treat," they'd say.

Gomer had a little treat at 6:00 am (baby's feeding), 8:00 am (owners' breakfast), 10:00 am (baby's feeding), noon (lunchtime for Mommy), 2:00 pm (baby's feeding), 4:00 pm (Mommy's coffee break), and 6:00 pm when all hell broke loose with the baby's feeding, the owners' dinner and the dog's meal of the day.

Gomer continued to chew well into the evening when the baby had another bottle and the adults enjoyed a snack. And if she was lucky, the baby would wake up during the night for another round of feeding. Gomer's meals tapered off as the little girl got on a regular schedule with only breakfast, lunch, dinner and a couple of cookie breaks a day. Then Mommy got pregnant again. At this point she decided Gomer couldn't tolerate the stress of another sibling, so she was put up for adoption where "she'd be the only baby."

Her new mistress, Grace, a compulsive overeater but average dog owner, brought her to a vet. He took one look at the four-year-old tub that weighed 29 pounds, and said, "She's grossly overweight. She should weigh no more than 17 pounds!" Well, Gomer went from feast to famine overnight, and spent the rest of her life looking puzzled.

Sure that the food went down Gomer's throat too quickly for her to taste, Grace tricked the dog by stretching the treats and halving the amounts. Instead of offering "Gome" one-half apple as a treat, that same apple served as two or more treats. Instead of rewarding her with one milk bone for a medium-sized dog, she gave Gome one-half of a milk bone for small dogs. She followed the vet's instructions and put her dog on a special reducing diet that afforded her more muscle than fat. By the time the dog pared down to 19 pounds, Grace was a wreck.

"Some day I'm gonna kill that damn dog. Every time I try to make dinner, she's there. Behind me, in front of me, between my legs. I'm afraid I'm going to trip over her and hurt her. Or kill myself."

The dog seemed to have ESP. She could be sleeping four rooms away from the kitchen. "You could hear her snoring!" But, whenever Grace opened the refrigerator door ever so quietly, the dog miraculously appeared. "The dog lives for food," she claimed. "But so do I. I belong to OA, and when I see how she approaches food it makes me feel very uncomfortable. I see myself in her. But, you know she helps me control both of us. I don't snack like I used to because I feel so guilty eating in front of her, and I won't overfeed her because I know it's not good for her."

But compulsive overeaters—people or pets—can be sneaky. "Gomer used to go to work with me. One morning, I stopped to get gas. In the time it took me to pump $7.50 worth, that dog managed to open my purse, take out my lunch, chew through a plastic bag, eat my corned beef sandwich and fall back to sleep. I shouldn't have been surprised," Grace said. "She had already learned how to yank open the cabinet door with her teeth, and get to her food that I had pre-packaged in individual servings. All the bags were in a plastic container with a tight lid. One night she had five dinners, the one I served her and the four she helped herself to."

Gomer went to the big kennel in the sky looking quite svelte. Had she resided with compulsive overeating owners who didn't recognize their problem, her fate would have been different because overweight people tend to have overweight dogs. As a food addict she would have eaten whenever they ate or whenever she begged for food, and she would have eaten herself to death long before her 15 years.

Sadly, when Dog-Gone Owners appreciate food too much, they enjoy it when their dog does, too. "It's sort of like Tubs bonded with me more than most dogs get attached to their people," said one client who was severely overweight. "Food made us inseparable." Tubs, who lived up to his name, always joined his mistress for meals or snacks, day time or night. "I guess you could say that eating is our favorite form of entertainment. The problem is," she giggled, "that we're getting too fat to get out of the house everyday."

Where Gomer and Tubs were hooked on food, Sandy, a Dachshund, was hooked on catnip more than the family cat. Periodically, Sandy would steal some of the catnip and get high, run around, growl, roll on her back and leap into the air. Then, she'd crash, lay flat on her stomach and sleep it off. The catnip didn't seem to hurt her any more than it hurt the cat, but usually dogs find something "better" to choose. Like . . .

Anything with sugar! Who says too much sugar doesn't affect people . . . or dogs? Think of owners who are addicted to candy, ice cream and cake, and chances are their dogs are addicted, too. The more the owner eats, the more the dog gets. The more the dog gets, the more hyper he becomes, particularly if he's hyperactive to begin with. When a dog wraps his lips around chocolate candy that contains caffeine and sugar, he can turn from a Dr. Jekyll to Mr. Hyde.

Snuffy, a wire-haired terrier, was always sweet and obedient except when he wanted to play and would become excited. One day his mistress noticed drastic changes in his behavior. "He's climbing the walls!" she told me. Shortly after this episode, the family went away for a couple of days and took Snuffy with them. "He was all right, but seemed a little jumpy to me." Back home, within four hours, he was climbing walls again.

After questioning his owners, I learned that Snuffy's favorite food was chocolate. When he was home, he ate it; when he was on vacation, he didn't, and he had symptoms of withdrawal. Back home, he got his fix again.

His owner hadn't realized that keeping chocolate candy in every room of the house was more temptation than addicted Snuffy could bear. Since she wanted to please him, it was normal for her to give him a piece of candy whenever he begged for one, several times a day. She thought Snuffy was on the honor system until she found him with his snout in a candy dish, helping himself. His craving had gotten the best of him. "Would you say 10 pieces of candy a day are too much for him?" she asked me.

"Only about 10 too many," I said.

The dog was able to de-tox when his owner emptied all the candy dishes and offered Snuffy sweets that didn't contain chocolate and caffeine.

Snuffy loved his chocolates, but another dog, Pepper, found his caffeine in cola. He'd simply lap a glass clean or empty an open can. "He just loves it when we entertain," his mistress said. "When it's party time, Pepper drinks Coke or Pepsi out of his own glass. I put a straw in the glass and he loves to chew it, but so far he hasn't learned how to sip through it."

When a pet becomes addicted it's generally a matter of "doggy see, doggy do." They simply imitate their owners who can't bear to remind the dogs they are dogs. This was the case with Julius who proved my conviction that there's a direct correlation between boozing couch potatoes and inebriated dogs.

Julius was the only pet in a household where he dictated the house rules. He had dinner with his owners. He sat on his own chair and ate people food out of his own plate. He slept in his owners' bed with his head on his own pillow. And before bedtime every night, he hopped up on the sofa with his master to watch one sporting event after another and drink beer. "He's partial to Miller's Lite," said his master.

"Why are you telling me that you encourage your dog to get drunk? Do you expect me to approve? I certainly don't."

"Ah, come on, Doc, he really loves it. And how much can one beer hurt him?"

"Enough to give him a hangover," I said.

"His is nothing compared to mine," his intelligent owner responded.

I have to admit, however, that Julius' drinking in his own home was preferable to his making the rounds of neighborhood bars, like Spud. Spud's owner, Amos, was told by his teetotaler wife that if he dared to bring any alcoholic beverage into the house she'd kill him. "And I mean it. If he wants to drink he can get out of the house to do it." So, he did. Once or twice a week he'd go to the tavern with his ol' drinking buddy, Spud.

Amos would buy one beer, ask the bartender for a saucer, pour an ounce or two of the brew into the saucer and put it on the floor for Spud. "When Spud's with me he entertains everyone who's in the bar. They like to see a drunk dog." The patrons would buy Amos a few rounds and when they tired of the floor show, Spud and Amos went on to the next bar. And the next.

I saw Spud one morning after his bar-hopping when Amos and his wife, Etta, brought the dog in for his regular checkup. "Amos did it again," she said through clenched teeth, glaring at her husband. "Took Spud to the bar. Got him drunk again."

Spud looked anything but hung-over. His vigorously wagging tail thumped the examination table and when he put his paws on my shoulder his eyes were bright, clear and alert. If that dog was suffering from too much booze, so was I.

"Amos, how much does Spud really drink?" I asked.

"Not much," he answered sheepishly.

"How much is not much?"

"Most of it ends up on the floor. But guys who have been in the bar are too far gone to notice how much he drinks because he acts real drunk."

"He doesn't get drunk?!" Etta asked.

"No, he just pretends that he is," I replied. "He likes the attention and he knows his behavior pleases Amos, but he probably doesn't like the taste of beer."

Other dogs, however, are genuine lushes.

Homer Basset was addicted. His drinking started as a gag when he got curious about the "cold one" his owner, Ben, enjoyed every evening after work. Homer begged for a taste. Ben wet his finger with beer and allowed the dog to lick it. Homer begged for more, and Ben poured a little into his food dish. Homer drank all of it, begged for more, and got it. Soon Homer was wobbling and stumbling around, and his owner thought it was very funny. So did house guests. It wasn't long before Homer drank and tied one on every evening.

Eventually Ben realized that Homer had developed a bad habit, and he tried to cut him off "cold turkey." The dog didn't appreciate this deprivation, especially since his master was still chug-a-lugging. He barked and howled until he, too, got his beer. If Ben refused to pour him one, Homer would deliberately and systematically set out to destroy the house. He chewed the carpeting and the furniture legs. He left calling cards on the bathroom rug. When he was reprimanded for this bad behavior, he lifted his leg and urinated on his master who then thought it was time for a veterinarian consultation.

I suggested that Ben switch Homer from the real stuff to a non-alcoholic beer. That didn't work. He didn't like the taste of it, and he seemed to know there was no alcohol in it. Homer wanted his nightly "fix."

"Offer Homer regular beer that you dilute with a little water." Ben called the next day to report, "He drank it. Didn't seem to notice any difference."

"Great. Tonight add more water to the same amount of beer and each day increase the water."

That seemed to work for about a week. Then Ben called again.

"I think I added too much water."

"What makes you say that?"

"Homer turned up his nose at his beer, walked into my closet and peed on my shoes."

"Good point. Decrease the water."

That night Ben got out a few shot glasses, an eyedropper, a glass of water, a bottle of beer, a roll of masking tape and a marking pen. He mixed various strengths of beer and water in each shot glass, marked the ratios, and then held a "taste and tell" party for Homer. He offered each sample to Homer, starting with the weakest blend. "Man, was he ticked off! First he just ignored the shot glass I held under his nose. Then he began to growl and glare at me. Finally, I offered him a sample that he could smell, and he drank that. Now I know how much it takes to keep him happy."

Happy and hooked.

Yes, alcohol can be a problem to dogs. And to average owners, too, who are sabotaged by people who feel that any dog . . . even one that doesn't belong to them . . . is fair game.

Vicky, a client, said she made the mistake of telling a friend that her tiny poodle was a sneaky party drinker. "Doodlebug likes to empty the glasses after the guests leave," Vicky whispered. At Vicky's next gathering, the same person slipped the dog a Bloody Mary but didn't think it was worth mentioning. Fortunately, another guest tattled on her. After the party ended, Doodlebug began to bump into walls and trip over his feet. Then he passed out. His owner was so alarmed she called the rescue squad, and told them to come with a stomach pump. But "when they found out the victim was a drunk dog, they told me to call my vet. So I'm calling you. And then I'm calling my so-called friend and telling her to keep her paws off my dog!"

I assured her the poodle would be fine after he slept it off. Sure enough, the next afternoon he was well on his way to recovery, a little groggy and unsteady on his feet, but at least he was on his feet. I later heard that Doodlebug never got near tomato juice again.

The number of alcoholic dogs I encountered in my practice far exceeded the doped dogs. That made sense because then and still now it's more common for people to admit they legally partake of liquor than to confess they illegally smoke pot, snort coke, take LSD or inject heroin.

Speaking of these drugs, one user admitted giving his pet LSD. When he heard his pet howl and saw him turn over on his back he rationalized that the dog was enjoying himself. "I wanted his dreams and fantasies to come true, like mine do when I'm on a good trip."

Most owners who are fond of drugs don't treat their pets to the hard stuff. However, since many consider marijuana to be recreational and harmless they don't think twice about blowing smoke in the animal's face. The end result is that there are probably as many dogs that have developed an affinity for marijuana as there are those that prefer booze.

According to Su-zee's owner, the dog is a doper because she likes the smell and taste of marijuana. Whenever her mistress indulged, Su-zee cuddled as closely as possible, stuck her nose near her owner's mouth and inhaled deeply when her mistress exhaled. If she saw a joint on the coffee table, she picked one end up with her teeth and moved her mouth up and down as if she was trying to puff, and she'd even eat some of it. Su-zee's owner saw no harm in allowing the dog to get high once in a while. "I swear," she said, "the dog gets so relaxed and happy she looks like she's smiling."

What made this revelation more interesting to me was that Su-Zee's owner was a widow in her late 60s who said she had been introduced to grass by her 72-year-old lover. "There's nothing like a little pot to get you in the lovin' mood," she said. I'll have to take her word for it.

I have often wondered what owners were thinking of, indeed what planet they were on, when they decided to go to these extremes with their pets introducing them to overeating, alcoholism and dope. Yet I can understand why. Food, beer and booze, and grass can be and are enjoyed by people, and in moderation pose no great hazards. Combine that thought with the owner's philosophy of "what's good for me is good for my dog" and it's logical that these people want to share everything they like with their pets. But I was convinced there were Dog-Gone Owners who lack the common sense to think, "I weigh 125 pounds, my dog weighs 30 pounds, maybe he can't tolerate the same type or amount as I can."

I ran across only one case where both the mistress and family dog had insomnia and were addicted to sleeping pills. Alice chalked hers up to constant worrying about her dog, Shaggy. And Shaggy's was a result of puppy distemper that left her with leg tremors. After several years, when Shaggy's symptoms disappeared, Alice tried to stop feeding her a pill every evening. But by then, the dog was hooked to the pill and the nightly ritual where the "ladies" got together to ensure their sweet dreams.

I suggested we give Shaggy a substitute of sugar pills to see if they'd relieve her emotional dependence on drugs. Alice's husband came to the clinic to pick them up. "Alice's doctor wants her off her damn pills, too," he said. "She tries, but after three to four nights of walking the floors she starts taking them again."

He paused. "You know the pills look alike, and we have a lot of the dog's pills left over. Do you think we could play switcheroo?"

"Like giving Alice Shaggy's old pills? It's worth a try. The dosage is so small they can't hurt her."

Shaggy was able to sleep, thanks to her placebos, Alice took her dog's pills "so they wouldn't go to waste," and after a few nights she adjusted to the minimal dosage. Then she decided to switch to sugar pills. "I have to set a good example so she won't get addicted again," Alice said. The last I heard, the "ladies" were drug free and sleeping like proverbial tops.

But only a few stories have a happy ending where addictions are concerned. One instance of this is Dolly's Dilemma.

Dolly decided on the advice of her physician to stop smoking. Soon after this, her dog, Fritz, began to act jittery and whine. Neither a dog psychologist nor I could determine the reason for his behavior. Dolly was nervous enough as a result of nicotine withdrawal from her usual two packs per day, but she became more nervous worrying about Fritz.

One day she thought she'd jump out of her skin watching Fritz suffer. Out of desperation she retrieved a crumpled pack of cigarettes from a hiding place. "I kept a few in case of an emergency, and by God, this was an emergency!"

As soon as she lit up, Fritz planted himself on her stomach and sniffed the smoke. For a few hours he simmered down and acted normally. Then he began to act up again. Dolly lit up again, and again Fritz calmed down.

Dolly resumed smoking. "Who do I listen to?" she asked me. "Whose health should I worry about? Mine or the dog's?" Being a Dog-Gone Owner, she opted for Fritz.

After seeing dozens of addicted dogs, thanks mainly to their owners, it was anticlimactic when Wendy came in with her English sheepdog, complaining that Duchess was addicted to television.

"Watching TV is all she likes to do. She loves to see people on the boob tube. But she turns into a maniac when an animal appears on the screen."

"What do you mean?"

"She charges the TV set. Hits it with her muzzle. Look," she said, prying open her pet's mouth, "she chipped three teeth trying to bite the animals."

A muzzle solved that problem. Before Wendy and her husband turned on the set they muzzled the dog. Her husband watched his favorite westerns, Wendy viewed her nature shows, and Duchess still attacked the animals but couldn't chip more teeth.

If a dog must become addicted to something, I heartily recommend TV.

It's truly the lesser of the evils unless you own a dog like Duchess. Dog psychologists, however, feel that for sensitive dogs more than three hours of TV per day tends to make the pets agitated. Generally the worst that can happen is that their pets will become hooked on particular programs.

One client insisted his dog, Fella, was so addicted that he picked up the remote control with his teeth, pushed the "on" button' with his paw and flipped through the channels until he was lucky enough to catch his favorite—rock music shows. "He has taste in his arse," said this owner.

Another client told me she walked into her den and found her two dogs, three neighborhood dogs and two visiting cats watching "Mr. Ed." The animals supposedly "horsed around" the same time every week to catch the show. (See illustration 18.)

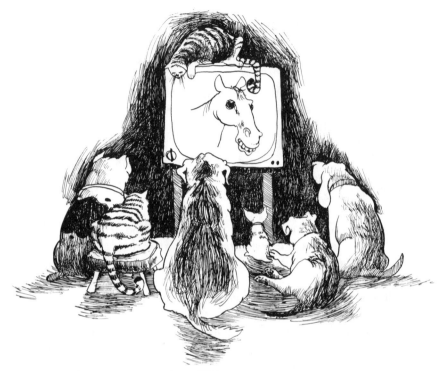

18. Watching Mr. Ed on TV

More than once I've heard clients say that television, rather than creating problems put an end to them. Pierre, a French poodle, stopped destroying slippers, sock, shoes, curtains, drapes and rugs the day his owners forgot to turn off the TV before they left for work. That afternoon when his mistress returned home from her part-time job, she found no tatters or shreds. From then on, the set stayed on. More times than not, Pierre was so engrossed in his soap opera that he hardly took the time to greet his favorite person. (See illustration 19.)

Speaking of soaps, I've heard that there's a new one called, "Take All My Children To Another World For As The World

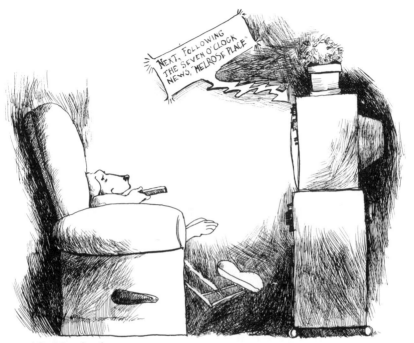

19. Hooked on soap operas

Turns I Have Another Life To Live. Or, maybe it's called "All My Puppies," or "As The Fleas Turn I Have Another Itch To Scratch." Who knows? Maybe the canine couch potatoes will get lucky, and one of these days they'll get so bored reviewing yesterday's happenings and wading through all those commercials that they'll fall asleep and avoid addiction altogether. If not, contact a few Dog-Gone Owners and put A-DUTI in their ear.

Chapter 6

Sometimes Mother Nature Needs A Helping Hand

I was in my clinic holding a pair of dangling gold earrings, looking at an overweight Beagle with a bent tail and listening to her owner, a harassed divorced woman with two daughters, two jobs and one runaway ex.

The woman wanted to confer with me about piercing the dog's ears. "She's one of my girls. The others have pierced ears. Bessie wants them, too."

She leaned closer and whispered, "She's so bowlegged a dachshund ran between her legs, and she frets over her tail constantly trying to make it stand straight. She knows she's no beauty, especially after she watched the American Kennel Club special on TV. She's depressed. She's overeating to compensate for her defects. Now, if we let her wear earrings she'll think she's attractive. She needs them."

I pointed out that Bessie's earrings could get wet when she drank water or sniffed around outside, and might also attract food and insects like magnets.

"Look, Dr. Vine, I detract from the bump on my chin by accentuating my eyes. You have to make Bessie's ears the focal points to detract attention from her tail and legs. The holes don't have to be down low. Pierce her ears higher."

"The rings could catch on objects and tear her ears."

"I'll exchange the wires for small studs with posts."

"They could infect her ears."

"Just pierce one. I'll use an antibiotic on her ear and the post. We'll take our chances."

I sent her home to talk with Bessie and get her final opinion.

Good heavens, here was another request from a Dog-Gone Owner to improve on Mother Nature. Where would it end?

I thought of the era of pioneers and homesteaders. Dogs were then as they are now companions for the elderly, playmates for the young and security for the isolated or the frightened. But back then dogs also served a more vital purpose. They worked. They helped the shepherd confine his flock. They fetched wild birds the hunter shot down for food. They guarded the home and family at night against thieves, murderers, and wild animals. Those dogs worked like dogs, as hard as their owners.

I don't recall reading that any of our busy ancestors in scrambling for day to day survival . . . like Bessie's mistress . . . spent a second of their precious time discussing the necessity of piercing a dog's ears. "Sometime, Pa, between milkin' cows, churnin' butter, feedin' chickens, plowin' the back 40, and puttin' up a new barn we're takin' Ugly Dawg to that vet man, Dr. Goody, to git her ears ready for Grandma's opals."

Dawg saw the veterinarian only when he had a major problem, like four broken legs or a pitchfork wedged down his throat. Dawg took care of some of his own problems, such as eating grass when his stomach was upset. His owners handled other problems by relying on folk medicine or leaving it to Mother Nature to decide his outcome. Dawg recovered or he died, and that was that. If Dawg was ugly, that created no problem because that's the way he was meant to be.

Times are different now. For starters, dog owners, especially extreme owners, monitor their pets' state of body, mind and soul closer than their own, and take their pets to a veterinarian more often than they themselves go to a doctor. But clinic visits for checkups, inoculations or treatments often screen another reason for an appointment: owners believe they have to give Mother Nature a helping hand.

For example, it's routine to crop the tails and ears of Doberman puppies so their looks conform to specific standards that were established for competitive show purposes. Ironically, even if a Dobie's owner doesn't intend to show him, he'll still be cropped. It is more ironic that some quirky owners fix what isn't broken in the show dog though he should be presented with the appearance, gait, musculature and teeth that Mother Nature gave him.

A fact of show life not widely advertised is that some owners have subjected their pets to enough cosmetic surgery to make human beings envious. We're talking "show biz" that involves travel, time, inconvenience and great expense to owners. "You have to give your dog an even chance when he's in the ring," more than one owner of champions told me, "or else don't bother to enter him."

Despite this belief, very few show dogs have been radically altered. But, as in every area of life, there are always those people who will find a way to increase their competitive odds. For a few owners, an "even chance" means they had their show dogs' teeth straightened or capped. Or perhaps they had their crossed eyes aligned, or their third eyelids removed so their eyes didn't protrude. Or maybe they had their overslung or underslung jaws corrected, their sagging breasts reduced or their missing testicles replaced with soft prostheses. Given this tiny bit of assistance maybe doggy will rise head and tail above his relatives and at least win an honorable mention, if not the best in show or breed.

How ethical is this practice? The feeling among more unscrupulous owners is "what judges don't know won't hurt them." Just as people shop around for a surgical genius to correct their flaws, the whispered word gets around that Dr. Miracle is the best man or Dr. Wonder has never failed. That means you don't take your pet in need of cosmetic surgery to the nearest veterinarian who cured Sassy Poodle's flea problem. You find the specialist.

The counterpart of Dr. Goody, the old time vet who made house calls and treated a wide assortment of ills, is still around today. Like his counterpart, the family doctor, the veterinary general practitioner is becoming less common. Increasingly, veterinarians are certified specialists, paralleling people doctors. At last count I came up with about 25, enough to carry a dog from womb to tomb.

One new client who used the services of several doctors for herself and her family confessed relief after her dog's first visit to me. She thought I'd overcharge her to examine Bootsy before referring her to a hodgepodge of "expensive" specialists to treat each of the dog's problems. After the visit she was only too happy to pay the bill. "In one fell swoop you prescribed a diet for Bootsy, expressed her anal glands, treated the rash on her back, diagnosed her arthritis and pulled her abscessed tooth. "You're a dietician/proctologist/dermatologist/rheumatologist/dentist—five specialists rolled into one!"

Specialization in veterinary medicine was inevitable. The knowledge and expertise were there, the resources were available, and the impetus was spurred on by the desire of dog owners who want the best for their four-legged loved ones.

So now, you don't have to settle for an ordinary vet. You can take your pregnant bitches to an obstetrician; pups to a pediatrician, and old timers to the geriatrician. Canine tooth problems? There are dentists, orthodontists and exodontists. Who else? There are dieticians, gynecologists, urologists, metabolists, endocrinologists and internists. Chiropractors, orthopedists, surgeons and neurosurgeons. Cardiologists. Oncologists. Roentgenologists. Pathologists.

For most dog owners this list is too long. "Veterinary attention, love and good care are all a pet needs."

"Oh yeah?" says the extreme owner. "What about Binky's psychological welfare?" The list grows.

Today veterinarians are trained and certified in animal psychology and animal behavior. Supposedly they're for the dog that has deep personality conflicts, traumas or unacceptable behavior; however I suspect they're more for the owner who wants an immediate cure for Whoozer's unexplained depression or nervousness, and a valid explanation why he "isn't his good old happy self." If these specialists can't appease the owner, there's still hope because . . .

The list goes on.

Animal psychics are available to communicate with the dog and pinpoint a problem. "It was really something to witness," said one owner. "The psychic asked Oliver if she had permission to speak to him, and he said she did. Then she held his head in her hands and explained to me she was sending him images and he'd send some back to her. After a few minutes she told me Oliver was lonely because he's alone all day. He wanted a playmate." He got one.

There are also animal psychic healers. They diagnose pup's problem and through hands-on treatment alleviate or correct it. Sometimes, according to these healers, they're helped by the spirit of doctors "from the other side."

But some owners who believe in things parapsychological don't take their dogs to psychics or psychic healers. They feel they don't have to. They're blessed with the same talents.

"There's no question that my dog and I communicate," Bertha told me. "I know exactly what's going through his mind. Remember I thought my dog had an allergy because he was chewing the hair off his legs? Well, he straightened me out when I telepathically asked him what his problem was. He told me he was afraid of the dark because he had nightmares that he had chains around his legs and he was locked up in a dark barn. We think it was a past life regression. He told me to leave a night light on. I did, and now he's fine."

In this new age there's much emphasis on self-healing, holistic wellness, and the connection between body and mind to restore and maintain balance, harmony, serenity. No conscientious owner ignores these for his or her pet when they're available out there. Goodie! More specialists.

One of my clients, Emma, brought Nonny in because the German Shepherd was in great pain. The old girl had a herniated disc that was inoperable due to her age and the risks. I felt she wouldn't survive surgery, and sadly told Emma that short of prescribing pain medication and hot packs there was nothing I could do, except put the dog to sleep.

In Ugly Dawg's time, he might have been retired to spend his days lazing in the soothing sun until Mother Nature said, "It's time to go." Not so today.

"Dog doo! I won't put her to sleep and I don't accept that my Nonny has to suffer until she dies naturally. I'm taking her to my acupuncturist," Emma said.

She called to report that after 15 minutes of having the needles inserted Nonny stopped crying, lifted her head for the first time in months, and took a nap. She was fine and we were happy. Considering my traditional medical training, I was also a little surprised.

In those days, we veterinarians were leery of unconventional and alternative therapies that supplemented or replaced traditional treatment, even when the results were beneficial. But people change with time, and today most of us accept acupuncture as a valuable treatment for various conditions. One vet friend said, "I willingly refer patients to acupuncture specialists. It often helps when traditional methods don't. I go for the needles, too; they help my crappy back a lot. That forces me to keep an open mind."

Personally, I didn't knock the "unusual" therapies, but I didn't understand them. I felt the same way about them as I do my computer. I don't know how it works or why it works, but it works when I want it to. And it's a darned sight better than my old manual typewriter.

Admittedly, I straddled the fence, but it allowed me to see the good on both sides. "If it helps, it helps. End of argument."

So, it didn't take much for me to recommend alternative measures to clients, among them doggy massage to relax their pets, reduce their muscular tension and relieve their aching arthritis. "Be sensible about massaging your dog, though. Do not, under any circumstances, overdo it," I'd tell them.

Unfortunately, I neglected to tell this to Yolanda. She couldn't understand why her Pekingese backed away and whimpered whenever she saw her mistress briskly warm up her hands before each treatment.

"How often are you treating Ralph?"

"Oh, as often as I get a chance," she said.

"How many times a day?"

"Oh, about six to seven."

"Forty to 49 times a week?"

"About. Do you think that's enough?"

"How long do the treatments last?"

"About 30 to 45 minutes. Do you think I'm doing it enough? Long enough?"

Then she mentioned she Rolfed Ralph because she heard from a friend of a friend that Rolfing worked wonders for her and her Malamute's aches and pains. The results may be beneficial but the workout is anything but tender touches and gentle pressure. I've known 200 pound men who admitted they cried during treatment. Enlightenment hit Yolanda like a ton of kibble. "Rolfing is ruining Ralph!" she gasped.

Yolanda developed the touch of an angel, limited massage to once or twice a day for 15 to 30 minutes, and Ralph looked forward to his back rubs.

The more my clients benefited from alternative treatments for themselves, the more they felt it necessary to combine alternative with conventional treatments for their pets. New age words peppered reports from my clients.

"We took Talbert to have his meridians cleansed."

"Floppy has a blocked third chakra."

"Tippy's aura shows she is agitated!"

Meridians? Chakra? Aura? I didn't know what these people were talking about so I asked a young friend to enlighten me.

"Simply put, Lou, meridians are highways running through your body, making way for 'chi' or the body's vital force that give you pep and good health," he said. "Sometimes there are traffic jams in the meridians. Find the chi entrance and exit ramps in the meridians, apply pressure at the right spots to break up or clean out the jams, and chi travels on. Understand?" He didn't wait for me to answer before he continued.

"Aura. An energy field around your body. Made up of seven energy centers or chakras that correspond to different areas of your body. Sometimes a person's aura gets imbalanced or opens and leaks energy; when it's undercharged, it causes illness or disease. A trained healer 'reads' or analyzes the aura. He balances, repairs or charges it through various therapies to correct what's amiss in the body. Get it?" Clear as chocolate pudding. But if it works, it works . . . like my computer.

The new age certainly added zest to my practice. I couldn't wait to hear from my clients who treated themselves and their dogs at home. Which discipline did they experiment with? How did it affect the people? How did the dog respond physically and emotionally? Did the clients see any changes in the dogs?

Owners who practiced meditation tried to involve the dogs. "I turn off the phone, bring Bo into a darkened bedroom, and repeat my mantra," Dora told me.

"How does he react?"

"He's having a little trouble. At first his right ear jerked whenever he heard me chant. I say it more quietly now. But he refuses to concentrate. I think his mind wanders until he falls asleep."

The meditation lulu was a client who was a most unpleasant person. Sarcastic, snippy and intolerant, rumor had it that she had alienated husband, grown children, friends and even her pastor. I know I felt like popping her one whenever I saw her in the clinic because she'd yank Pudgy Pug's leash and snarl, "Move it, you damned lazy dog."

Then suddenly I was looking at a different woman who was tender and loving toward her pet. She'd pat Pudgy, scratch her ears and kiss the pug on her mouth. I was eager to find out what caused this wonderful change and wanted to ask,

"How come you stopped acting like a rotten wretch?" Instead I said, "Things seem different now. Better."

She confided she had finally realized she had problems and she wanted to change. She started going to a psychologist who, after a few weeks of therapy, suggested daily meditation to expand her awareness and encourage non-critical thinking. During one meditative period she went into an altered state of consciousness unlike any other she had experienced. "It was beautiful. Blissful. I rode a glorious rainbow that undulated ever so gently as it carried me to paradise." She then described paradise, and her unexpected encounter with God. "Just for a second, but it was long enough for me to know that I'd better change my ways, love my Pudgy and be good to her." On her way out of the examination room she turned to me, and said, "Did I mention that God was in the form of a dog?"

Who am I to comment on that remark? I just know I liked the outcome.

Another client went the route of warm whirlpool baths, incense, candles and spiritual Indian music to create the desired ambiance for her and her terrier. "It works for me; it should work for Judy, but it doesn't. She starts coughing and growling the second she walks into the bathroom. I think it could be the incense." Eliminating the scent ended the cough but the growling didn't stop until Judy's owner replaced the Indian chants with Bruce Springsteen.

One of my favorite stories involved a tiny and elderly client who brought in her 15-year old cocker spaniel. Miss Lucy said she was alive at 89 and had big plans to celebrate "the big one-zero-zero" because reflexology (massaging her hands and fingers and feet and toes) eased the pains in her knees and head and kept her insides as clean as a whistle.

"I'm an old woman who's feels like she's coming apart at the seams," she told me, "but I'm still here. And what's good for this old cocker," she added, pointing to herself and then her dog, "is good for that old cocker."

Miss Lucy showed me how she treated her dog. "See, I get in real good between her toes on all her four feet. When she yips . . . like this . . . I know I found a sore spot. When she nips me . . . like this . . . I know I better stop."

Now let's discuss medicines.

In Ugly Dawg's day people didn't pop pills like crazy because there weren't many pills to pop. They remedied ills with folk medicines like vinegar, honey, herbs, dandelion and peppermint teas, mustard plasters, poultices, liquor and good old chicken soup. They were the guinea pigs: If it worked for them they commonly used it on their animals.

Then came technology, research and development, and the tables turned. Animals were used to test people medicines. If it didn't kill the test animals, it was judged safe for human beings. Now, in a sense, veterinary medicine is back to square one where owner Joe is the final test animal for pet Jocko.

I prescribed drugs for animals that had been proven effective for humans. If they didn't kill people I knew they were safe to use on my patients. I liked that.

The muscle relaxant Valium was one such drug. So were hormones, such as Depoprevera; the old Micky Finn sleeping pills; antibiotics, such as penicillin; and antidepressants, including Prozac, which has become the drug of the '90s.

Given the correct veterinary dosage, anything from major drugs to baby aspirin or Kaopectate can work wonders for a troubled or sick pet. Problems arise, however, when owners blindly feed their wonder meds to their pets.

Kate continually fought what she called "the battle of bumper hips." She did this, she said, by weighing herself three times a day, starving herself one to two days a week, and swallowing an assortment of pills she got from a "fabulous" diet doctor.

Kate had brought in Brandy, a grossly overweight terrier who panted for breath. I instructed Kate to stop feeding her pet people leftovers from the breakfast table, the lunch table, the dinner table and the TV snack tray.

"Gosh, that means I'll have leftovers on my plate, tempting me and driving Brandy crazy."

"Throw them down the garbage disposal."

Kate nodded her head and went home with Brandy.

The next time I saw the dog I had a hard time believing it was the same terrier. Brandy was emaciated, and so nervous she jumped at every sound.

"How's her weight now?" Kate asked, with a gleam in her eye. "You can't complain that she's overweight."

"On the contrary. She's much too thin. What have you been feeding her?"

"Only her regular meals."

"Nothing else?"

"Well, I didn't like the idea of punishing her by denying her leftovers. I came up with a kinder idea."

"Which is . . .?"

"Well, I had a bunch of extra diet pills so I put one tiny pill on her plate." I gasped when she told me the name of the drug. The tiny pill that Brandy chowed down every day contained an "upper," an amphetamine strong enough to drive some people into the psychiatric ward. (See illustration 20.)

Bizarre as this may sound, it's not unusual. Unthinking owners—too many of them—have fed their dogs the same narcotics and sedatives, the same uppers and downers, the same vitamins, prescription drugs and over the counter medications that they take. After all, a cold is a cold, insomnia is insomnia,

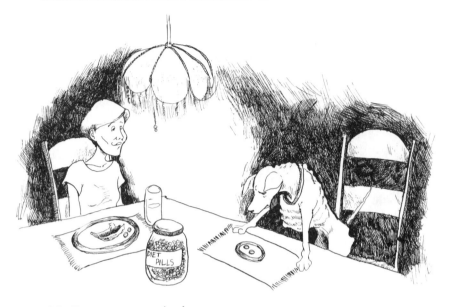

20. Dog on owner's diet

nervousness is nervousness, obesity is obesity, et cetera. When dogs aren't dogs but people, what harm can there be in giving them people pills?

A lot. But try convincing a Dog-Gone Owner.

In many cases the pets don't need people pills. They don't need dog pills, either. They simply need to be left alone—in Mother Nature's hands.

One owner who considered himself a medical whiz was greatly concerned about his dog's constipation. Not content with my suggestion to stop feeding his dog so many bones, he created a unique remedy. "One of those fiber pills mashed up in prune juice." Then he called to report "Petunia is pooping all over the place!" What could I suggest to bind her?

"First you gave her dynamite. Now you want cement. How about stopping those fiber pills?"

"Doesn't she need some kind of pill?"

"NO, she doesn't," I roared.

But when there are pills around the house, there is often temptation to medicate the dogs.

Robert E. Lee Schnauzer had an appointment for blood tests. His mistress had noticed that the dog bled too much and too long if he got a small cut. Tests proved negative for hemophilia and parasites in the blood, so there had to be another reason.

"Robert E. Lee doesn't need this on top of his migraines," Miriam said.

"Migraines?" I asked.

"Excruciating. He rubs his head with his paws and moans and wipes his face on the carpet. Poor baby. But . . . "

"Let me guess," I said. "You give him adult aspirins and they stop his migraines."

"Right."

I explained that aspirin caused the bleeding from the treatment he didn't need for the headaches he didn't get. "He's moaning because he enjoys rubbing his eyes and his face."

"He'll be fine? Honestly?"

It took a lot of talking to convince Miriam that Robert E. Lee didn't have migraines, glaucoma, detached retinas or a few dozen imagined conditions. In this respect, she was the same as other owners who suffer through non-existent medical crises with their pets.

"What's wrong with my baby?" is a question clients have asked a few million times during my practice. Too often the problems, if any, were caused by a master or mistress blinded by love. They sensed something was wrong, usually a past or present problem they had experienced first hand, and they found the remedy in their medicine cabinet. Unless they were believers in "the more natural, the better."

Many people avoid man-made drugs with a passion. They find their remedies in health stores, buying homeopathic drugs based on natural herbs and products. Need I say that what goes for them goes for their dogs?

So, when Alphie came to see me, suffering from a raging rash, I knew his owner had already treated him with an assortment of salves and over the counter preparations. I prescribed cortisone.

"Cortisone?" Alphie's daddy shouted. "That's a steroid!"

"Yes. He needs it."

"No cortisone!"

"What would you do for yourself if you tried everything and nothing worked? Refuse your doctor's suggestion of cortisone that would stop the terrible itching and burning? Be sensible," I chided.

"I'd kill myself before I used any of that toxic stuff."

"Hold on a minute," I told him as I started to walk out of the room. "I'll see if I can find a gun so you can shoot Alphie."

Alphie got the steroid and his rash disappeared. "I guess drugs are OK," his owner later admitted. They're more than OK when they're appropriate for the dog and the problem.

But, a word to the wise. If, by some chance, your female dog decides to get sexy, do not feed her birth control pills. Those people pills don't work on dogs.

Now it's not only in the previous areas that owners feel they have to help Mother Nature keep their pets in tip-top form. Let's talk about cleanliness. That's a subject that seems to occupy the minds of many owners.

We are a brain-washed society, taught to believe that any natural body odor is an affront to anyone within smelling distance. As we've all heard, and many of us believe, cleanliness is next to godliness. According to Dog-Gone Owners this means that dogs should not smell like dogs. Every orifice and hair on their precious bodies should be a balm to our noses, like essence of roses. However, Mother Nature with her fine sense of humor endowed dogs with an "aroma." Sometimes it's pleasant; other times it will bowl you over.

Mighty few are the people who tell an owner, "Your dog stinks." First, if you dared say that, your friendship probably would end abruptly. That's the same thing as telling a friend, "You know, I've been meaning to tell you for years that your breath would kill a moose."

Secondly, most pets of Dog-Gone Owners do not stink because they're as clean as their owners. Some are cleaner. That was the case with a man who had a horrid case of body odor but blamed it on his dog. "Sunny smells bad," he told me, "like something crawled up his rear end and died."

I didn't know how to tell the gentleman that he, not Sunny, was the stinker. "Hummm," I said, as I tried to find a tactful solution, "let me think about this for a minute. Hummm. Hey, maybe this will work. I don't know what kind of deodorant you use, but I suggest a spray-on. O.K.? Good. Now, after your nightly shower, and after you spray on the deodorant, just rub what's left around the hole of the dispenser on Sunny. Don't squirt the bottle, though. He only needs a tiny dab of the stuff." Sunny's B.O. disappeared.

Thirdly, if an extreme owner gets the slightest whiff of a bad smell emanating from his or her dog, he or she will get to the bottom of it and immediately eliminate it. This can be good and it can be bad. The negative side is that over-conscientious owners will kill or mask a dog's odor that helps a veterinarian make a medical diagnosis. On the positive side, these folks have perfected the act of sniffing.

More than one client has held a dog to my nose . . . or pushed me toward a dog that was too large to hold . . . and said, "Dr. Vine, smell him! He has a weird, faint odor. Smell it?'' Most times I couldn't because the dog didn't smell bad. His owner just had super-sniffing ability. However, once I recognized the odor of decaying salami that I found trapped between the dog's cheek and teeth.

I don't object to people using soaps, shampoos, antiperspirants, tooth pastes and mouth washes. Actually, the closer I get to the users, the more my appreciation grows. But I believe these products are for people, not pets.

Most of my exceptional clients don't agree. Often they told me, as if I had never heard it, "If it's good for me, it's good for my dog."

I could have taken odds that dogs brought to the clinic for a general checkup had at least been bathed within 24 hours. If I didn't compliment the appearance of my fastidious patients quickly enough, owners said, "Betty Boop has to smell good for Dr. Vine," or "Fritzie just came from the beauty parlor." In so many words they were telling me that their dog was so clean I could eat off his paws or back. That's the way it should be; that's the way it is. That was their interpretation. It was not mine.

I believe owners too often go overboard in their determination to deodorize and sanitize their pets. Had owners settled for giving their pets a "Saturday night bath" with a dog shampoo, I wouldn't have objected.

"Really, Marsha," I told one client who had bragged about her dog's cleanliness, "it's all right to take Corkie into the shower with you, but not every morning. And, you have to stop lathering him up with a people shampoo for fine limp hair." (See illustration 21.)

"I might as well change brands," she moaned, "it isn't doing much of anything. Anyway I don't think he likes it, because he tries to scratch it out."

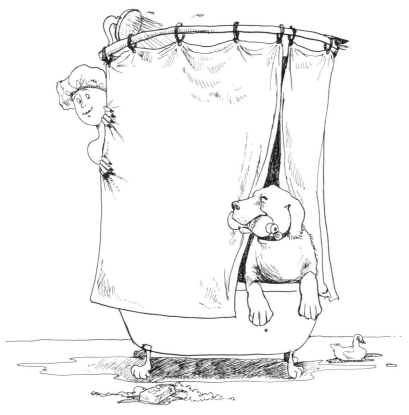

21. Showering together

"He's scratching because it makes him itch. The shampoo dried out his skin."

"Nah. He's just disappointed that his hair isn't thicker."

Marsha finally agreed to limit the co-ed showers and shampoos to one a week, promising, "And I'll stick to a dog shampoo, too." She liked the results so much she began to use it on herself. "It's great! Feel my hair. It has body. It's clean. It smells good." That flip side of the coin is typical, following the tit-for-tat belief that "what's good for my dog is good for me."

If that sounds strange, consider that one popular shampoo and conditioner began as a product to groom horses until people tried it and adopted it. And, let's not forget the salve that's used on cow udders and teats to keep them soft is also used by people to treat their chapped, roughened hands.

The bulk of my remarkable clients used dog shampoo on their pets, but finding the "right" brand often created a problem. Did the dog like the scent? Was it easy to rinse out? Did it turn his coat into a work of art? Did it cleanse, eradicate fleas and moisturize the dog's skin until it was as soft as a baby's bottom?

"You know," said one woman, "using the same shampoo week after week isn't the best thing, no matter what you say. We have several. When it's bath time, Spookie reaches into the cabinet and takes out the one he wants."

Most of my far out clients had daily grooming schedules for their pets, which was fine with me and for the dog. They brushed their dogs' coats daily, wiped food off their face and dirt off their paws, and tidied up bottoms that the dogs neglected. But I had clients who went overboard.

A few cleaned their dog's nails every evening. "Well, mine get dirty and I don't take off my shoes, drop down on all fours and walk through poo-land. Besides, she needs her nail polish touched up every night and you can't paint over dirt."

Others flossed the dog's teeth after meals. "You know how irritating it is when meat get stuck between your teeth," one woman reprimanded, after I told her it was unnecessary. "What do you do? Ignore it? Fat chance!"

Dozens brushed their dogs' teeth, even if the dogs ran when they knew what was coming. "I don't care what Daffodil says," an owner said, "I drag her out from where she's hiding.

I'm her daddy, I say what goes, and we don't go to bed without brushing for three minutes.''

Wiping the dog's bottom after walks was religiously done by many vigilant owners even when the dog only urinated. "It cuts down the smell," Vanessa said. "It's not that Will isn't interested in personal hygiene; he's just in a hurry to play."

One Dog-Gone Owner in particular stands out because she spent so much time grooming her dog I wondered when she had time for herself.

"I brush Baby Bro's teeth after every meal. Then I brush his hair and use an aspirator on his little nose. After walks I cleanse his wee-wee and his tushie with diaper wipes, and wash his feet with soap and dry them. After meals I wash and dry his face. And, every night I give him a bath, towel dry him first, then use a brush and a blowdryer, and spray his favorite perfume on him, Chanel No. 5, to finish.''

"What? You don't spray his pits with deodorant?" I kidded her.

"It never occurred to me," she said. "We'll start doing that, too."

I bluntly told her she better not. We were talking about a dog, I reminded her, not a person. She replied indignantly, "I've never heard such unkind words in my entire life."

Striving for external cleanliness wasn't enough for many owners. They had to take internal matters into consideration. For example, dogs were not supposed to create and expel gas. I didn't know this until a client told me I had to give her dog an enema. "You have to do it," she said, "because Sam's tooting up a storm. Even he can't stand the smell. I gotta do something!" His owner and I waited for Sam to perform. Nothing happened until he stood, stretched and emitted a tiny "toot" that I would not have detected had the dog not sniffed with interest.

"See?" his mistress exclaimed, "Look how he's twitching his nose in disgust. I told you he was very gassy!" I said we should be as lucky as Sam, and sent them home with some charcoal pills . . . to give to Sam when his flatulence becomes excessive. The first eight don't count."

All signs of a healthy digestive track bothered an extreme owner, and I heard about it. "His tummy rumbles. It shouldn't, should it?" "She burped three times yesterday. Maybe I should change her diet." About the only unusual client who took normal digestive sounds in stride was the owner of an old dog that always sounded like a whoopie cushion. Ziggy's explosions never bothered her because she never wore her hearing aid.

Speaking of innards makes me think about the woman who talked about giving her dog a douche. "Douche?" I asked incredulously. She nodded her head. "Have you tried giving her one yet?" She shook her head. Times like that made me grateful for life's mini-blessings.

She leaned forward and whispered, "But she'd feel so much fresher after her periods." I was most thankful she asked me about it before she subjected Queenie to one.

I knew that if I didn't nip this subject in the bud, she would have asked me to recommend one for Queenie—vinegar, herb scented or God knows what else that was available in those days. It would have been a waste of time to get into a debate in which she insisted it was the proper "womanly" thing for Queenie while I insisted it was totally unnecessary. She dropped that idea after I told her she couldn't use a people nozzle on the dog and I didn't know where she could purchase one sized for a schnauzer.

For the most part the dogs, all the way from tiny to huge, tolerated the rigors my unconventional clients put them through. But some rebelled. For years Gina lavished daily attention on Tiny, an immense mastiff. She massaged and manicured him. She washed and dried every inch of him. She pampered and perfumed him. She played chants and lit incense for his spiritual well-being. Tiny voiced his objections through soft "wuffs" and moans that grew louder as time passed. "He doesn't appreciate what I go through for him," Gina complained.

Then one day she returned home from a shopping trip and thought a hurricane had ripped through her bedroom and bathroom. "I think Tiny went over the brink! He chewed my spiritual tapes, ripped my how-to books, ground the incense to powder, clawed open bathroom cabinets that held his grooming products and bit through plastic bottles. Goop was everywhere! The only things he didn't destroy were his comb and brush. I cried, and the wretch sat there and wagged his tail."

Aha, wise Mother Nature got in the last word after all.

Chapter 7

Lifestyles Of The Rich And Infamous

As a veterinarian I have seen the similarities and differences between a Dog-Gone Owner on a limited income and one with unlimited finances. Both love their pets, care for them above and beyond the call of duty, and are as generous as possible.

For example, in the same week two clients showed me new collars they had purchased for their poodles. Mrs. Brown said she found Peter's in a discount store, "on a pegboard hook I almost passed by." Mrs. Carter, on the other hand, mentioned, "I consigned a jeweler to create this diamond-studded original for Pierre." Both owners were equally happy because their baby had something new to wear. Price didn't matter.

But let's face facts. The more money Dog-Gone Owners have to spend for their dogs to have the better things in life, the more they spend.

Owners on budgets paid to have their dogs' healthy teeth cleaned or their decaying teeth pulled. "What other options does Dickens have?" Few, since years ago cleaning and pulling were standard procedures.

Yet, wealthy owners balked at having pet's teeth extracted insisting on the same options they had. "John Boy is not going to walk around with gaps in his mouth," Mrs. Previn adamantly told me when I suggested pulling one of John Boy's front teeth. I sent her to a veterinary dental specialist who made the dog a false tooth.

Another owner convinced an orthodontist to make braces to straighten her dog's crooked teeth. "Why not? It's possible. If I'm willing to pay for it, pay for anything, what's the big deal?"

"Sometimes it makes me feel guilty," one client told me, "because when my children were little they had to do without. We didn't have money for luxuries. We barely made ends meet. Now we have money, the kids are financially secure adults, so we tend to indulge Buster."

Buster was nearly blind and couldn't hear very well but he led a dog's life that was privileged. He had a color TV in his private bedroom, slept on a king-sized bed, wore personalized clothes, had a Cabbage Patch doll as a best buddy, and enough toys to distribute to several animals and children and still have plenty left for himself. For his 15th birthday, because "Buster looks forward to car rides every day," his owners bought the dog a new Cadillac. "It's a worth while investment," his dad said, "because Buster loves it. He even chose the color. We went to the agency after hours, and Buster picked out what he wanted."

That owner, however, couldn't keep up with the Joneses. Sam and Melissa Jones, that is. This wealthy couple took their two St. Bernard dogs with them wherever they traveled. They only thing that was a bit unusual was that instead of riding in their owners' convertible, the "boys" were chauffeur driven in their own air-conditioned station wagon. Since the caravan has been all over the United States, you may have seen them.

A local celebrity in my area was Jean Paul, a toy poodle, who visited the clinic weekly for an allergy shot. Folks were rather sarcastic when they saw the uniformed limousine driver pull into the parking lot, lift Jean Paul off his large silk pillow on the back seat and carry him into the clinic. "My, my, aren't we fancy?" one client in the waiting room remarked.

"Forget fancy. It ticks me off that his mother is too busy to bring the dog in herself. Honestly, some people . . ." said another.

Often, Dog-Gone Owners invest in items they believe will keep their pets happy. This was especially important when these clients checked their dogs into my boarding kennel.

Mrs. Chapman had told me, "Rene gets lonely staying in a private boarding run here, and that greatly concerns me." I had an inkling how much it bothered her since "how to best minimize Rene's separation anxiety" was the sole subject I could count on her to bring up before she took off on one of her frequent trips.

"I don't want him to pine away. Should I leave something I've worn but not washed . . . even though the thought of that makes my stomach turn? Or a pair of shoes? I know I should do something." Between you and me, Rene was a happy dog as long as he had contact with any person, but I couldn't share this with Mrs. Chapman, Rene's "sole and beloved companion."

She solved her problem by commissioning an artist to paint her portrait. Then she had her butler/chauffeur bring the custom framed canvas to the kennel along with Rene. "This will help him when we're apart. I would have had his portrait painted, too, but that would have been too bulky to travel with. So I just take along a few 8" X 10" professional photographs." (See illustration 22)

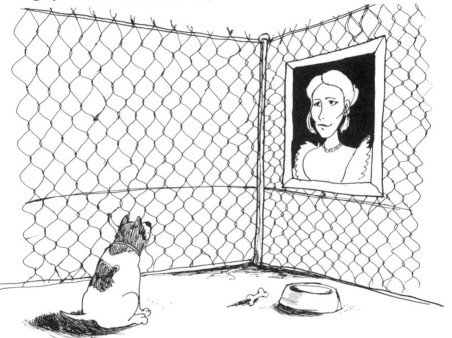

22. Out of sight—out of mind

Several clients bought radios so their dogs could listen to soothing music or talk shows. Mrs. Dunne went a step farther by buying a TV to put in her dog's run so he could watch his favorite programs. "Here's a list of the hour and day of the programs. Follow it exactly, please, because I don't want him to watch trash." Since Mrs. Dunne frequently traveled, she left the TV at the kennel, "with the understanding that when Bingo is a guest he has exclusive use of it."

Mrs. Foster paid to have her retriever Rocky's cast iron bathtub toted to and from the kennel via a trucking service. "Rocky doesn't like the new plastic pools you have here," she explained to me. "He insists on swimming in his own tub." We found room for it.

However, when Mrs. Foster and Rocky went to New York each year they left his tub at home. "Too much trouble making plans to transport it." At the same time she didn't want Rocky to worry about where his tub was. "And when I have to get away for a weekend to relax from life's stresses, I don't want him to worry about me, either." Mrs. Foster averted both emotional problems by checking Rocky into a luxury kennel in the Big Apple. "I ordered the works for him. He was kept busy most of the day so I don't think he missed his tub, but I'm sure he was miserable for me the entire time."

She described the chauffeur-driven limousine service to the puppy palace, the air-conditioned and plush carpeted suite complete with piped-in music and large color TV. I heard about the three gourmet meals a day, the sauna and the massage room, the whirlpool bath, the dog treadmill and the salon that pampered the pets with baths, manicures and grooming sessions. (See illustration 23)

"I imagine Rocky fared quite well," I mentioned.

"I hope you're right," she said, shaking her head. "So far he hasn't complained, but separations are very traumatic."

I think it's more traumatic for kennel owners who rashly promise to provide their boarders with whatever they're used to having at home. Many of my clients had established daily rituals for their dogs that were easy to fill, but unusual. One took her spoiled Dalmatian to a bar for a glass of beer. Another spiked her mongrel's morning milk with exactly 20 drops of brandy. A third rocked his beagle to sleep in his arms while he sang a lullaby. I went along with these requests. But

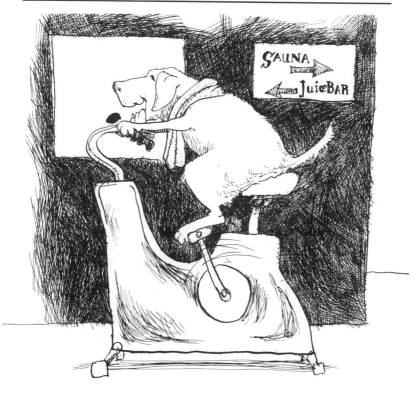

23. Dog Health Spa

when an owner asked me to allow his Scottie to sleep in my house, between my wife and me, I drew the line.

"Why won't you accommodate me, Dr. Vine?"

"Because I'm a one dog man; I only sleep with my dog."

The owner who almost nudged me into a new career was Mrs. Sullivan.

Mrs. Sullivan traveled more than most people. When she went to Europe, she called every day at five minutes before eleven our time, no matter where she was and ask for a progress report on Dove.

"Don't leave out a detail. Tell me what he had for breakfast and dinner. Did he eat it all? Reluctantly or eagerly? Did he go potty? How often? How much? Did it look healthy? Who took him for a walk? Did he behave? Does he miss me? Did he cry?" After she was reassured he was fine, she'd demand, "Doctor, kindly put the phone to Dove's ear so he can hear mommy's voice." (See illustration 24)

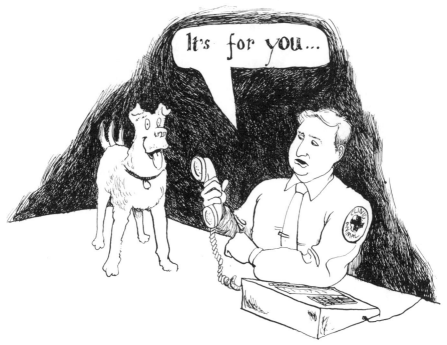

24. Daily phone calls

A call a day was tolerable. Not welcome, but tolerable, if the client and patient I had to ignore during the call were understanding. But when she traveled in the states, where "long-distance calls are the same as calling around the corner," she'd ring me morning, noon and afternoon, asking to speak to both Dove and me. The time I wasted dropping what I was doing to talk to her was minimal compared to the aggravation I felt because I could not convince Mrs. Sullivan that Dove never heard a word his mommy whispered into the phone. Dove was stone deaf.

It always interested my staff and me to see what indulgent owners brought to the kennel to accompany their dogs. "Luvie" or a dog's favorite belonging, was common. Clients by the dozen brought pillows and blankets and toys. Some were K-Mart quality while others screamed Bloomingdale's. Food and water bowls were commonplace, too, and ranged from dented stainless steel to personalized china. "He won't eat anything if he doesn't have his bowls," I'd hear. Yet, it's odd that when owners forgot them, and I convinced them not to make a trip home to retrieve them, especially if they had to catch a plane, the dogs managed to inhale their food from my bowls and still wag their tails.

On occasion, we came across some interesting items. Once we unpacked a bottle of perfume for Sheba who "can't fall asleep unless you put a dab on her ears and front paws." We received a bottle of creme de cocoa for Minny Pin who "has to unwind mid-afternoon." And, we opened a monogrammed suitcase that contained enough Orville Redenbocker popcorn, popped and bagged in individual servings, to satisfy a huge movie theater filled with people. "Heidi has very discriminating taste," her owner informed me, "and munches only the finest."

One day, while unpacking the over-sized suitcases a Dog-Gone Owner of two schnauzers sent in with her dogs, an attendant said, "Look at this. Four goose down pillow that are thicker than my mattress. Why four pillows for two dogs?"

"She said they destroy them very quickly, and if the twins couldn't go to bed with fluffy pillows they'd stay awake all night," I explained.

"The price tags are still attached. They cost $199 each. She spent close to $800 for pillows?"

"No, she told me she bought six pillows in Florida. Some place in Palm Beach. She spent over $1200."

"I'm going to faint! Here's more. Two hand-knit blankets appliqued with a pattern of dogs. Each one has the dog's name knitted in the border. And, oh my God, two pairs of shorty pajamas. I guess if it were winter we'd find sleepers with attached feet. Think she'd adopt me? I want to be one of her dogs!"

I, too, benefitted from wealthy clients. Frequently my receptionist joked, "Lou, it must be that time of the month again," as she handed me a floral arrangement, or a gift-wrapped box that contained candy, watches or trinkets of all kinds. Each gift came from the same rich woman and was accompanied by a hand-written note supposedly written by her Bichone Frise. Had the note not expressed Jacque's appreciation for my veterinary services, I might have gotten the wrong idea. Well, it has been documented that more women fall in love with their veterinarians then with their own doctors. In this case, alas, it was simply gratitude.

"It's pleasant to have money. It's more fun to have it today than it was twenty or thirty years ago," one client from the old days recently told me. "There are hundreds of dog things I can buy for Lulu and Lawrence."

"Like what?"

"There's a treat machine where the kids can get their snacks by pressing down a bone shaped handle. It sort of looks like an old gumball machine. That was dirt cheap. Only 30 bucks. I got them matching bomber jackets, too. I never would have thought of that until I saw an ad for one made of waterproof imitation leather and a synthetic lambskin collar. Only $30, each. But, my kids are used to the real thing, so I had my dressmaker make two using genuine leather and lambskin."

"They cost a little more?"

"Well, only about $300 each, plus the cost of the materials."

"A mere pittance," I joked.

"I can't take it with me. I've got it, I spend it."

Wealthy Dog-Gone Owners not only spend it, they spend it in ways that don't occur to most dog owners. I was around animals for 40 years, and during that time I talked to thousands of owners. I'm still around my dog and I'm still talking to owners. But today when I hear what lengths generous owners go to make their pets happy . . . in other words, make themselves happy . . . I occasionally still raise an eyebrow. Who would have thought?

I know owners who take their dogs to chiropractors or acupuncturists every week. And others who treat their dogs to a weekly massage. "What good does one visit do? A weekly visit is preventative therapy. Costly? Yes. So?"

So, it's not as costly as sending a disturbed dog to Denmark for private psychiatric therapy. "We tried everything we could in the United States. We had no choice." This owner chartered a private jet to fly her and her neurotic dog there and back, and she stayed in a four star hotel for a month. "I was a little surprised at how much I spent, but it was only about $5000 more than I anticipated." (See illustration 25)

At times, an abundance of money complicated issues. If, for example, Mrs. Lord had owned only one home and called

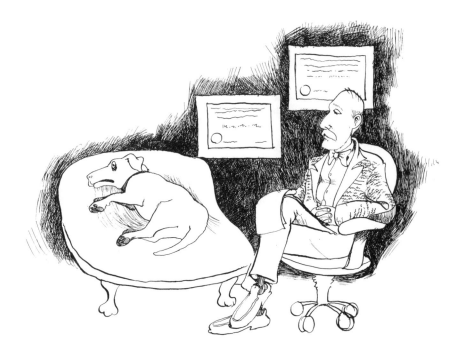

25. Dog shrink

me to make a house call, I would have been minutes away. However, Mrs. Lord was in her vacation home in the Bahamas when she phoned one morning about 5:00 am.

"I need you now, Lou," she sobbed into the telephone. Her poodle was very ill. She had taken Chanel to a veterinarian who had diagnosed an ear problem but didn't know how to treat it. The dog was dying. "You specialize in ears, Lou, you'll know what to do."

Within three hours Mrs. Lord's private plane arrived in North Carolina to pick me up and fly me to the Bahamas. By the time I arrived at her house, Chanel was in terrible shape.

Examination pointed to a tumor in the dog's middle ear. Immediate surgery was indicated. But where would we do it? Where could I find the surgical instruments I needed?

Mrs. Lord swooped up the dog, said, "I know where, let's go!" and we ran to her car. She broke the speed limit driving to a local hospital . . . for people . . . where she screeched to a halt in front of the entrance. We raced inside with the dog, bypassing sick people on our way, and dashed to the hospital administrator's office.

Not once did Mrs. Lord remind the administrator of her annual multi-million dollar endowment to the hospital, but minutes later I was in an operating room with assisting nurses and an anesthesiologist.

Once I removed the tumors and saw that the dog suffered no complications, he returned home to recuperate, and I was on my way back to North Carolina in the private plane. I spent the flight time wondering what the administrator would have replied had Mrs. Lord told him she insisted that her dog recuperate in a private room of the hospital. I doubt if she would have heard an argument.

As recently as ten years ago, euthanasia was standard treatment for sick, aging or injured animals. Owners tended to go along with it because they considered it humane. "Why should Pixie suffer any longer? Do it, Doctor, put her to sleep and give her peace."

While I know several wealthy Dog-Gone Owners who agreed to euthanasia, many more didn't. If they could pay any amount of money, wasn't surgery worth a try? Even experimental or dangerous surgery? Yes, it might kill the dog; however, it might alleviate or remove the dog's pain, give him a few more good years and, in the case of cosmetic surgery, make him look more attractive.

Having ample money allowed these people to endorse any treatment for their pets that was known to man. When I'd outline their options, my suggestions and the possible results, I'd repeatedly hear, "If it helps, let's do it now. You can tell me how much it costs later."

One of my clients owned a 15-year-old beagle that showed common signs of old age. Chloe had warts and skin tumors, and her few remaining teeth were abscessed or badly in need of cleaning. Those were her minor problems. During her examination, I saw a huge mass blocking one of her ear openings. I couldn't determine its size, but having seen it in other dogs, I knew it was cancer. Removing it meant major surgery, including a radical resection of the ear canal.

It was possible the cancer had spread into vital organs where it could not be totally removed; it could be a type that spread quickly or one that didn't respond to treatment. "There are many questions I can't answer until we test or I subject her to surgery. And the old girl might not survive such extensive surgery."

Chloe's mistress and master were in tears. They knew something was wrong with her ear but thought it was the same fungus that had plagued her since her puppy days. They weren't prepared to hear that she had cancer.

"Go home and think about what you want to do," I gently suggested, mentioning again that euthanasia was one solution to Chloe's problems.

They looked at each other, and the husband said, "There's nothing to think about." His wife nodded her head, and added. "Right. You have to operate."

I outlined the approximate costs for treating each and every condition, and added fees for biopsies for all tumors, several complete blood work-ups, anesthesia, X-rays, antibiotics, intravenous catheters and fluids. The last expense I estimated was "possible radiation treatments or chemotherapy, which-ever is indicated. For that I'll line up an oncologist friend who treats people."

They didn't flinch at the expense that was to come. They simply told me to go ahead. "Let's see how well she tolerates minor surgery. Start with the small lumps on her rear because they're minor and work up to her ear, because that's the worst."

Over the next few weeks Chloe and I saw a lot of each other. I'd operate, and after a short stay she'd go home to recuperate. Another week or so, another procedure. Because of her advanced years and general condition, she was at risk each time I anesthetized her. Much to her owners' relief and mine, she survived every ordeal, including the ear resection.

After she healed, I referred her to a colleague who adminis-tered chemotherapy at his people clinic after hours. "Let's keep it our secret, Lou," he said. "Only you, the owners, the dog and I will know. I don't want word to get out that I had a dog as a patient."

What Chloe's family paid for her medical attention from beginning to end was enough to cover the cost of a luxury cruise for two to Europe. In the thank-you note I received from her owners, they wrote, "We thank God every day that we can afford what so many unfortunate people cannot."

Money makes the world turn around, as the saying goes. I'd like to add that to Dog-Gone Owners like Chanel's and Chloe's, money also opens doors that are sealed more se-curely than Fort Knox is to you and me.

I was visiting a wealthy friend when he awoke me early one Sunday morning by loudly knocking on the bedroom door. Through the closed door I heard Frank say in a terrified voice, "Shadow has been trying to have her puppies all night, and she's in terrible pain. Please, Lou, do something. Help her."

I opened the door to see tears running down his cheeks as he held the Scottish terrier in his arms.

After examining Shadow I realized that one of the pups struggling to be born was in a breech position. I couldn't move or turn it. "A Caesarean operation is the only way to save her and the puppies."

"Well then, go ahead and operate," he urged.

"I can't." I was facing the same problem I had with Mrs. Lord. "I don't have instruments, and we can't operate in the house."

He called the head surgeon at the local human hospital. "Get the operating room ready. My dog needs a Caesarean. I'm leaving the house now with my dog and her doctor." Two seconds later he slammed down the phone, and turned to me. "He told me to come right in. The hospital is at my disposal."

Of course it was. Frank was the hospital's best benefactor, donating a fortune each year.

When we arrived, two doctors and four nurses were waiting in the readied operating room. While I scrubbed down, the anesthesiologist put Shadow to sleep, and attendants shaved and prepped her abdomen.

Within minutes and with no problems, six pups entered the world. I held up the last one, and said, "Meet the little trouble maker that blocked the path for himself and his siblings."

"Lou, you're holding Lou. That's what I'm naming him."

"You hate it when people name their dog people names. You said you'd never do it."

"True. But this time is an exception. You deserve the honor, and I have a damned good reason for doing it. I didn't want to lose Shadow. The puppies are wonderful, but they're a bonus. It's Shadow that means everything to me."

As far as I know, Robin Leach has not yet interviewed Frank. He should. But first he should get in touch with Perry Deluxe.

Perry, a multi-millionaire, lived to work, make money and share his wealth. Similar to others in an enviable financial situation, he was most generous to his family and favorite charities. Perry thought nothing of donating millions of dollars here or there, wherever he saw a need or desire that money could satisfy.

One of Perry's pet charities was taking in abandoned or abused dogs and providing for them on his grounds. He would have moved them into his house, along with the two companion dogs, Luke and Matthew, that ate and slept with him and followed him everywhere, but his current wife objected. But by the time the dog count hit 27, Perry and his fourth or fifth wife had divorced, and he was fed up with his disappointing children. He turned all his love and devotion to his dogs.

He scheduled a meeting with an architect, an engineer and me to design a luxury dwelling worthy of his foundlings. "I want it directly behind my house. Build it, and build it right," Perry insisted, with an imported unlit cigar clamped between his teeth. We team members listened for an entire evening as he said, "I want . . ." "The dogs need . . ." "Remember to . . ." "Don't forget . . ." As we reeled out of his house, the last thing he threw at us was, "Money is no object."

The "doghouse," as Perry called it, was a dream come true to any Dog-Gone Owner. Architecturally it duplicated some of the finer features of Perry's house, a southern mansion. The roof, the columns in the front, the window shapes and main entry were almost carbon copies, just a touch less ornate. The landscaping was magnificent, with huge trees shading the front, sides and back play yard of the elongated U-shaped dog house, with not a weed in the dense green grass carpet. Pavers covered the walkway between Perry's and the dogs' house and the path to the entry door. When you looked at the place, you thought you were walking up to a luxury one story hotel. The only thing missing was a doorman.

In the doghouse, the dormitory wing at the front consisted of 25 individual and relatively soundproof rooms, each designated for a certain dog. To ensure that everyone knew who was in which room, the dog's name was painted on the door and his or her medical chart hung above it. Perry's dogs eventually learned to walk on water, as his theory was that the dogs needed waterbeds for their comfort and health. Each room had piped-in music, "for soothing songs to keep my dogs calm," and a 15" TV set for broadcast and closed circuit programs. "I want them to watch animal and nature tapes. It's good for them!" And, of course, the rooms had a door leading to a private outdoor run that was covered by a roof. "Fresh air. They need lots of fresh air!"

The runs also had back gates that released singly or together at the push of a button, permitting the dogs to socialize in a large enclosed pen. The finishing touch was strategically placed, low bushes along the far end. "Hell, fire hydrants would spoil the looks, but I want them to know where they should do their business."

Perry had instructed us to make sure "the runs will be easy to clean and keep the dogs' feet dry and comfortable." The builder installed an automatic timer to operate pressure cleaners, and embedded electric elements in the cement to dry the wet runs and keep the dogs' paws toasty in nippy weather.

Back inside, the kitchen ran along one side of the U-shaped structure. That room contained a dishwasher and sinks, stove, garbage disposal, refrigerator, ample cabinets and plenty of counter space. The room looked somewhat ordinary until you saw a huge walk-in freezer. "It has to be spacious. I'm filling it with prime cuts of beef, Grade-A poultry and special treats that a nice woman makes to order. I want a power generator back-up in case the power goes off. My dogs don't go hungry, and they sure as hell don't eat food that might have spoiled."

Next to the kitchen was the office. Here, a full time employee filed records, kept on top of veterinary and grooming schedules, acted as a buffer between Perry and his ex-wives and children, and informed Perry immediately if a dog seemed "a little off his feed."

On the opposite side of the U was the grooming room for Blondie, the professional groomer, who was on Perry's staff and on the premises five days a week. Half the room was designed for bathing the dogs. Cabinets loaded with plush towels of all sizes billowed out of open cabinets, and a jacuzzi bathtub with gold plated handles for the dogs' weekly baths sat in a corner. "Some dogs like water and love to swim everyday, and others need daily water therapy, so it has to be big and deep enough for my largest dogs." It was.

The other half was designated the "beauty parlor." Here, Monday through Fridays Blondie bathed, brushed and groomed the dogs, and regularly trimmed the long-haired dogs to keep them looking they way Perry wanted, "like they were born to this life." (See illustration 26) Blondie had told Perry what she needed, and Perry provided it. Shelves and cabinets held every imaginable product that could be used on a pampered dog. I saw toothpastes and toothbrushes, after-bath colognes, combs, brushes, scissors, clippers and a large mirror, too. "They have to see how nice they look; it's good for their self-esteem."

"Don't forget yourself, Lou," Perry had dictated. My hospital room was next to the grooming room. It was furnished and completely equipped like a veterinary hospital, including an X-ray and surgical unit. Perry didn't allow any of his dogs to leave home, so I performed every necessary type of medical procedure there. At least twice a month I'd make scheduled

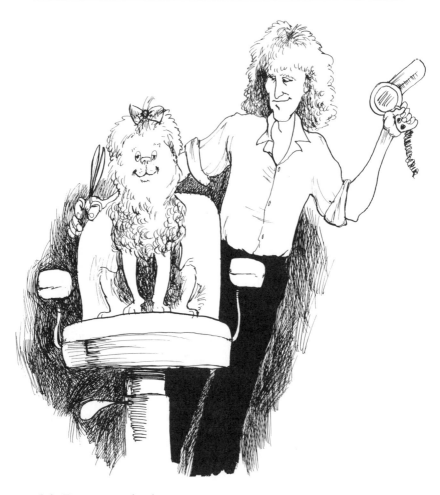

26. Beauty is the beast

house calls to examine the dogs and treat in-house any medical problems that arose. "If you need nurses or anesthetists, bring them in."

At completion, with the architect, engineer, builder and me in tow, Perry and his companion dogs walked from furnished room to furnished room, and personally tested each waterbed to assure themselves the comfort level was ideal. They checked every inch of the doghouse, a job that took most of one morning, while we peons held our breath. "What do you think boys," he asked, looking at his escorting dogs. "Good enough? I think so, too," he nodded. "Now, Lou, let's move my dogs in."

From that day on, Perry was a happy "daddy," as he assumed a goodly portion of the major daily chores of tending to his dogs. It wasn't different from the days when he had to cover a lot of outside ground, but it was much easier. More comfortable, too, because of the central air-conditioning system.

One of his kennel staff was the chef who handled everything from collecting and washing used food and water bowls to cooking the food, filling the bowls, loading them on a warming food cart and wheeling it to the dorm area. But Perry personally fed each dog.

"Lad's room," he'd tell the chef, holding out his hands for the food and water bowls. He'd go into Lad's room and close the door behind him. Perry went from door to door, took his time with each dog, and hand fed the finicky eaters. "It takes me hours," he told me, "because I give them as much undivided attention as they need. And some of them don't want their vitamins or heartworm pills, so I have to hide them in food or shove them down a couple of throats." If any dogs needed medications, he made sure they got them, too. Once he exited a room and rejoined his staffer, he updated the medical records on the door before he went to the next door. "Hours," he repeated, "but I don't mind because they look forward to our private visits."

Perry enjoyed pushing the button that released the run gates and watching his charges rush out to romp. "Look at them," he'd say with his eternal cigar, "are they having fun, or what? Hey you," he'd yell to an over-rambunctious dog, "cut that out or I'm sending you to your room!" If the dog didn't shape up, Perry marched into the yard, grabbed the dog and escorted him to his room. "Let me know when you're ready to behave," he'd growl, "and I'll let you out." Perry was one happy man, especially when he was on all fours, rough-housing with his appreciative roomers.

There was one section of his dog palace that made him unhappy though, the small cemetery that was set back to one side of the doghouse. "It's beautiful and serene," I told him, "with figurines and flowers. I like the benches you added, too."

"It's pretty enough, but I don't like it here. It doesn't matter which dog goes because they're all my favorites. I'll move a new dog into an empty room sooner or later, but I still feel like I buried a person. It hurts, Lou."

Perry commemorated each dog's passing with an engraved headstone made from imported marble that described their best traits. "Dover was a patient soul." "Here lies Reb, loyal to the end."

"Damn, I hate this part," he'd say. "I've got so much money, but it couldn't keep them alive, could it?" No, but he could pay to keep them in better health and alive longer than most Far Gone Owners could.

Many years ago Perry had an artist make metallic sculptures of a man smoking a cigar, with two dogs standing at his feet. The three figures overlook the dog cemetery. Eventually, the ashes of Perry, Luke and Matthew will rest in a concealed compartment in each figure. "We'll always be with our dogs.

They're a damned sight more my family than my ex-wives or my children."

There you have it. Lifestyles of several rich and infamous people who could not do enough for their dogs. But when you eye the bottom line, they were really no different from any other Dog-Gone Owner who enjoys spending money on pets.

Today, day care centers and exclusive sleep-away summer camps for dogs give people even more options. Shady's mistress can afford $5.00 a day or $20.00 a week to ensure hours crammed with dog fun while she's at work. "That's better than having her stay home alone all day, bored to tears. She socializes with other people and plays with dogs, and gets lots of attention. I would have loved to send her to summer camp, but it's too costly."

It was for her, but not for someone like Lacey Brown who calls it a bargain, "considering what Shotsy gets." Shotsy rides the private bus to camp, sleeps in his private room, lounges in his private patio, swims in the lake, goes on two walks a day, socializes with other campers, and chooses meals from the extensive menu. "If I wanted someone to hand feed him, they would. But he's a big boy."

How much does it cost to have a camper? You can figure in the neighborhood of $250 weekly for the basic luxuries.

"I pay a little more," Shotsy's mistress said, "because sometimes he wants an additional walk, or he needs a shampoo. Well," she admitted, looking a bit embarrassed, "maybe it costs me a lot more because I pay to have someone stay with him at night until he's asleep."

Lifestyles are all relative, and that brings us back to page one.

The more owners have to spend, the more they spend. But money or no money, all Dog-Gone Owners have one thing in common: their perspective is a mite off.

"Lou, that's a bunch of bull," one average owner sneered. "A mite off? If you were to ask a bunch of dog owners like me, we'd tell you the same thing. Those people who don't know what to do with their money except spend it on their dogs are so far out there you can't touch them."

"They couldn't care less."

"Ain't that the truth?" she concluded.

Chapter 8

Best Wishes For
Happy Occasions

A recent survey shows that 80% of United States and Canadian animal owners give their pets holiday and birthday gifts. I assume most of the recipients are dogs and cats, although birds, bunnies, pigs and horses probably would not turn beaks or snouts away from an edible present.

I expected the statistics to be higher. That's what I told a friend who dropped by to show me a holiday ad from a large pet market that amazed her. "Look at this," she said, pointing to the front cover. The words, "where pets are family," stood out like Rudolph Raindeer's nose. "There's even a page that lists 24—I counted them—last minute gifts for cats and dogs."

"What are you trying to say?" I asked her.

"It's ridiculous to put so much emphasis on pets."

"Them's fighting words to a lot of people I know."

"I don't care. I don't give my dog presents. Not even at Christmas. Especially at Christmas, for goodness sake. The idea never dropped into my head. I'm busy enough shopping for people gifts, cooking, cleaning the house, trimming the tree."

"Well, you're an average pet owner, and that's fine. But most of my clients are a little more enchanted with their pets than you are. So they buy them Christmas presents. They gift wrap them, too. Did you see this?" I asked her, showing her the part of the ad that touted reproducing the pet's photo as the family Christmas card. Naturally, the point was to have the dog wearing one of the festive articles the owner bought at the store.

"That's absurd."

"Maybe, but Christmas gifts are just the tip of the iceberg." Everyone's going to the dogs, including Hallmark."

"The greeting card company?" she asks. I nodded my head.

"Their latest line had 117 cards aimed at dog and cat lovers in categories like Get Well for the animal, Thank You for the vet and pet sitter, Congratulations to new owners, Sympathy to grieving owners, Happy Birthday to Fluffy and Fido . . ."

"And now more manufacturers and retailers can take advantage of all the animal nuts out there." She held up her hands, and said, "Don't tell me any more, please. I have enough to think about. I'm wondering if I should feel guilty because I don't feel guilty that I don't give my dog Christmas gifts."

If there is one season that affected my Dog-Gone Owners it is Christmas. As it approached, even the calmest of my clients became completely exhausted.

One November day a client called to say, "I've got a big problem, Dr. Vine." She sounded so upset that I suggested an office visit, and she charged in within the hour to unburden herself. "I do holiday shopping all year long, working from lists. The only family member who creates problems is Pansy. I've already brought her everything with a Christmas theme. Collars, leashes, clothes, toys, treats, a Christmas stocking . . . what's left?"

She vetoed my suggestion that she buy more of the same. "Can't. She likes variety." I suggested she knit her a sweater, a labor of love that Pansy would appreciate. "Already did, and she didn't appreciate it because she didn't like the neckline."

I didn't hit pay dirt until I sarcastically suggested, "Get Pansy her own Christmas tree."

The woman jumped up and kissed me. "What an excellent idea! I can lop off a few branches from our tree. Nobody will notice if I take it from the back. I'll trim them with doggie ornaments like chew sticks and milk bones tied on with ribbons and bows . . . . she'll love it!"

"There you go," I said, and there she went out the door, leaving me feeling smug. I had satisfied a minor problem for one client and could get to the major one of the next.

If Pansy's mom popped in today I could whip out that ad and say, "Hey, don't sweat it. There's an ample supply of gifts for pet owners like you."

There are leads and collars sporting Christmas motifs. There are rawhide "candy" canes, Christmas trees, wreaths and baskets, and antler headpieces. You can buy sleighbell collars, vinyl and fleece toys, sweaters and Santa costumes, bandanas that wish you a merry Xmas and that are embroidered with the pet's name. Need more? There are tree ornaments of a dog or bone personalized with a dog's name, and stockings stuffed with toys or treats or both. If you're willing to spend a few dollars, your pet will feel Santa paid him or her a visit.

Twenty or thirty years ago the selection was sparse in comparison. But then, too, it was equally important for Dog-Gone Owners to gift their pets. That was no easy task when there were such slim pickings in stores.

I saw one of my buddies pick up a dog collar, put it down, pick up another, put it down, pick up both and look at one and then another. And this was when leads didn't come in every color of the rainbow.

I tapped him on the shoulder and asked, "Need help, Alex?"

"God, am I happy you're here, Lou. I can't decide. Too many to choose from. If you were my corgi, which would you prefer?" He walked out buying both. "Yeah, I agree that the brown one would look better with his fur but I think he'd like the black one for dressy times."

"And why shouldn't I buy my dog presents?" an owner defensively asked. "Christmas is for pets, too. Primo knows Santa doesn't leave presents for bad kids. They're his reward for being a good boy all year. And," she glared, "don't think Primo doesn't expect them. I hide them and he always sniffs them out before Santa arrives. I've got to find a way around that."

After talking for a while she came up with her own solution. "Hey, maybe this year I'll wait until Christmas Eve before I rub a little beef fat on the outside of his gift wrap."

"Excellent," I agreed.

Part of the fun of buying dogs presents is giving them at the appropriate time, most often Christmas morning when the family is together. "If you don't think they're as excited as our other kids you've got another thought coming," said Primo's mommy.

"We take turns unwrapping the gifts," she said. So did a few dozen other Dog-Gone families. I found it hard to believe that dogs had the patience to wait until they got the go-ahead, especially if their gifts were "perfumed" with beef or chicken fat, but apparently they did.

"Carrie just sits there, smiling from jowl to jowl," my client Sara reported. "We know she's happy because she tap dances with her front paws and wags her tail. When we tell her it's her turn, she runs over to the tree and always picks out the right presents."

"Big whoop," said my friend Bob when I told him about Sara's dog. My Tuffy wears a Santa costume and delivers the gifts. Don't look surprised," he told me. "He knows who gets what. He fetches them from under the tree, one by one, and gives each one to the right person."

Did the pets get eggnog? "Of course." I can testify to that as I have treated numerous dogs suffering from Christmas Eggnog Sickness, also known as hang-overs. Did they eat breakfast with the family? Always. What's Christmas, unless everyone's at the table?"

If people who observe Christmas had difficulty and stress at holiday times, pity the Jewish people who observe Channukah. Tradition dictates that children receive eight gifts, one for each night of the holiday.

One client commented that she had wrapped the last of the Channukah gifts for her husband and three grown children—"only one per"— and her six grandchildren—"56."

"Hold on. Six times eight equals 48, not 56."

"You're not counting Chipster's presents. He gets eight, too. That last one was the killer. I couldn't decide what he'd like until I saw a large Star of David. I attached that to a new blue collar." She noticed a woman eavesdropping on our conversation. "Excuse me, Madam. Would you stop looking at me like I lost my marbles? Ignore her, Lou. Chipster is more excited about Channukah than my other kids. More appreciative, too. He's the only one that helps me with the potato pancakes," another tradition, "and cleaning up."

I visualized the dog wearing an apron and mixing the pancake batter with a wooden spoon. "He helps?"

"Sure, he licks all the plates clean before I put them in the dishwasher. And, as soon as the kids unwrap the presents each night, he drops the paper into a trash bag."

One of the traits I love about Dog-Gone Owners is that they have the capacity to truly enjoy life, unlike some sourpusses I could name. These owners have the gift of giving to others, often primarily their pets which can be unfortunate at times if it means they exclude people. But the giving is a source of joy except when it drives them up a wall.

"Life is a celebration," one of my earliest clients told me. "So, we celebrate all the usual occasions, and the personal ones that revolve around ourselves and our Fetcher, even far-fetched ones. Nothing makes me happier," she said.

She must have been in her glory when Fetcher lost his first baby tooth at the age of six months. She had a party for him. She had another when he graduated from obedience school. "I deserved it as much as he did, driving back and forth to school every week for months until he finally learned to listen . . . the third time around." And when he began to win prizes at dog shows, there were more celebrations. "Even if he doesn't win a ribbon, he has our love and respect. We want to show our appreciation, so we have parties."

Most Dog-Gone Owners wouldn't think of celebrating because Pup lost a baby tooth, graduated from school or appeared in a dog show. However, they have no trouble remembering and observing Pup's birthday. "My sister's birthday? I think it's April 14th or 15th. I have it written down someplace. Hiram's? June 19th. That was the first time I saw that precious tiny baby."

I received my poodle as a retirement present. I'd remember Maisie's birth date if I looked at her pedigree papers, but I can't recall where I put them. Or, if I thought hard and long I could come up with the month and the year I got her, and then I could count back eight weeks and arrive at an approximate birth date. This is not the attitude of a bonafide exceptional owner.

I probably would have lost business had I confessed to clients that our family didn't celebrate her birthday. Had I fibbed and said we patted her on her head, and sang, "Happy Birthday, Dear Maisie," I most likely would have seen many raised eyebrows, and heard, "What? That's all? And you're a vet?" Shame on me.

I realize it's the pleasure of outstanding owners to party it up for any occasion centered around their pets. After my early introduction to these devoted people, I occasionally imagined one looking at the calender and snapping to attention. "Oh, gosh, the ninth anniversary of Neptune's altering is next month. It's party time! Have to go into action! Invitations, decorations, menus, games!" My imagination, I later found out, actually underestimated how far a Dog-Gone Owner will go.

Leafing through the mail at my clinic one day I was happy to see that three envelopes didn't contain bills. They were invitations from clients to attend dog parties.

"After months of pregnant expectation, we're delighted to announce that Pipsqueak is finally weaned and now is officially ours. Please join us at our puppy's premiere appearance to celebrate her adoption into our family."

"It's Gonzo's fourth birthday! You're invited to his bash on Saturday afternoon! Treats for all. Gonzo says he doesn't want gifts but would appreciate a donation in his name to the animal shelter. P.S., people only this year. No pets, please."

"Mr. and Mrs. Franklin and Mr. and Mrs. Laurence are happy to announce the wedding of Moo-Goo and Woofer Sunday afternoon in the bride's back yard. Reception follows. Black tie optional but blue jeans O.K."

My wife and I accepted the first invitation, Pipsqueak's adoption bash. A tremendous sign plunked into the grassy front yard depicted a cartoon of a female puppy with a pink tie around its neck. Large letters in a deeper shade of pink declared, "It's a girl!" To make sure guests wouldn't forget Pipsqueak's sex, several pink helium filled balloons throughout the dining room and living room reminded us.

Pipsqueak's mommy, Mary, led us past the dining room table laden with pink petit fors, pink napkins imprinted with the dog's name, pink cups and plates with a puppy motif, pink champagne in an ice bucket and pink plastic champagne glasses.

"Come see the baby!" Mary whispered, touching her forefinger to her lips for quiet as she motioned to us to follow her into a hallway. Then pointed to a door hanger that cautioned, "SHH, Baby Sleeping," she ushered us into the bedroom where the little princess wearing a pink collar snoozed in a baby basket adorned with pink bows. After admiring Pipsqueak via smiles and sign language for a decent interval, we walked back into the dining room.

"How could we not celebrate her adoption?" Mrs. Smith asked, gazing at her husband who looked as if he wished he were anywhere else. "Right, honey?" Mr. Smith managed to smile. "We waited for her for such a long time." She turned to me and said, "You know I was at her delivery, didn't you?" I hadn't. "It was absolutely nerve wracking. And you have no idea how slowly time passes while you wait and wait until you can finally bring your baby home." The women in the room nodded their heads in agreement; most of the men shuffled their feet.

Mr. Smith muttered something about getting "this damned business over with we can get back to the ball game" and poured the bubbly. We drank a toast to Pipsqueak's good health and another to the lucky mommy and daddy, and admired the presents. When the men adjourned to the den, the women sat around the table listening to Mrs. Smith go on and on about the dog.

Mary escorted us to the front door when we left the party. "I'm just tickled pink you were with us today," she said sweetly.

Gonzo Bulldog's birthday parties were always affairs that guests talked about long after they ended because Gonzo's daddy owned a bakery and his mommy owned a craft shop. Are you getting the picture?

Each year the invitations were custom-made. Once we got an enlarged nose print with the words "I can smell my birthday is coming!" on the front cover. The following year they were of his enlarged paw print, "For the paws that refreshes, come to my birthday party." The next year a miniature outline of his huge rump told us, "I'm not fartin' around. Come or else!"

Peggy, Gonzo's owner, admitted she spent months planning his parties. "When he was a baby, it was easy. This year it was a problem because he vetoed everything I suggested. Then he found the solution. He insists that from now on we help his less fortunate brothers and sisters."

"Admirable," I said.

"You know it. But it's a challenge for us to follow through with the theme. I'm stumped by the invitations. How do we do donations to an animal shelter? Have dollar signs peppering the background, and in the foreground fat Gonzo pushing a wad of dollar bills over to a mangy, emaciated looking dog? That's tacky."

"I'm sure you'll come up with something unique."

They did. The invitations were heart shaped with a centered "furry" dog face. Bob made people and dog cookies shaped like fat bulldogs and skinny bulldogs. He made other cookies shaped like dog bones, dog bowls, dollar signs and hearts. He baked and iced a bulldog cake. His masterpiece, though, was cutting a cake into letters, frosting them, and arranging them to read GONZO THINKS YOU'RE GRAND TO GIVE HIS FRIENDS A HELPING HAND.

Peggy painted miniature dog bones on ribbons, and tied each around a rolled donation card from an animal shelter. She placed those in a basket, decorated, of course, with pictures of dogs.

At the party, Gonzo gave a kiss for each dollar donated to the cause. "Why couldn't they be chocolate?" griped one guest. "I hate it when a dog slobbers on you."

Guests ate, drank, endured Gonzo's kisses and his howling accompaniment to songs, and sat through his entire repertoire of tricks. "How do you feel about needy dogs, Gonzo?" He covered his head with his paws. "How do you ask for donations?" He sat up and begged. "What would you do if you collected a lot of money for the pet shelter?" He rolled over and wagged his tail.

As an encore, he was asked one more question whose response brought peals of laughter, "Would you rather be married or dead?" Gonzo immediately rolled over onto his back with his legs in the air, his eyes closed and his body immobile, as if he were in rigor mortis.

Invariably, Gonzo was the life of the party, his act-worthy of an Oscar-bringing many contributions from the audience.

Each guest took home a doggy bag for his or her pet that hadn't been invited to the party. "We didn't want to slight them, and they're probably upset because they weren't here,"

Bob explained, "but we didn't want a bunch of healthy happy dogs romping around. It would have taken the focus off the needy ones."

"It's a wonderful party," one guest remarked.

"Oh yeah?" retorted her husband. "I'm so happy I could lift my leg and pee. I could have lived without having that prune from the shelter show us a movie of abused and abandoned dogs."

At last report Gonzo changed his mind about his parties. "He was disappointed with the donations," Peggy said. "So he suggested we make a hefty family contribution instead of doing tons of work and spending so much money on a party. Now all he wants is to invite a few friends over."

Peggy was worried, though, because Gonzo had attended Duke's swanky birthday party. "Gonzo may regret that he didn't decide to have a fancy party, too. Duke fed his guests steak and kidney ragout served in china bowls, a shepherd's pie en croute and a liver mousse birthday cake. His mom had the meal catered, of course. But Duke is a snob, and Gonzo isn't, so I guess I don't have to fret about it."

My Maisie was invited to Gonzo's next party. The dogs sat around a table decorated with a birthday tablecloth, wore party hats, admired and tried to eat the birthday banners, and enjoyed the ice cream and bone shaped cake. They played "find the ringing phone" that had been hidden in a brown paper bag and seemed to enjoy that as much as "shred the toilet paper off the roll." (See illustration 27)

We adults played "Pin the tail on the cat," and helped by blowing out the candles, wiping a whiskered chin with a birthday napkin, and breaking the doggy pinata that had been filled with dog biscuits. A good time was had by all except when a few of the four legged guests tried to steal favors that didn't belong to them. While it was a fun afternoon, it made me

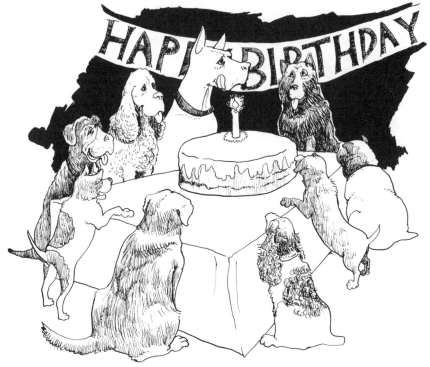

27. Dog Birthday Party

happy that Maisie was content to celebrate her day with no fanfare.

Weddings are joyous occasions for the majority of families, and certainly they're reason to celebrate, even when it's your dog that's getting hitched. Man or beast makes no difference. Dee said, "Hey, my niece looks like a dog and she had a big shindig. My schnauzer has better looks and morals. If anyone deserves a wedding party it's Moo Goo."

According to Dee, a dog wedding is ideal. "There's no sleeping around or living together before the ceremony. We know who our kid is marrying and we don't have to worry about having healthy grandchildren. The bride doesn't act like a prima donna and the groom doesn't tie one on at a stag party the night before. They don't drive us nuts demanding caviar at $2.50 a head, and the bride's maids don't bitch about their gowns.''

The weather on the wedding day was glorious, a good thing since the ceremony and reception were held outdoors. Guests wearing jeans or shorts coordinated with fancy blouses or formal jackets sat on lawn chairs, facing the gazebo. Uncle Mort from Colorado played ''Sunrise, Sunset'' on his accordion repeatedly until one guest said he was ready to barf and other guests told him to can it.

The bridal party was gussied up for the occasion. My Maisie was the bride's maid and wore a tulle skirt and sleeveless top; the best dog wore a black jacket and bow tie; and the flower dog had a bow in her hair and a basket handle clamped between her teeth.

They made it down the aisle, one after the other, without incident. It helped to have their owners call to them from the gazebo and immediately leash them. This was a smart move since Moo Goo was in heat and her virginity had to remain intact despite the best dog who lusted for her bod and was making no bones about it.

Moo Goo and Woofer were as attractive as any two chows could be. They were dressed formally, she in a white gown and veil, he in a tux and hat. Woofer was the epitome of dignity as he walked down the aisle, even when he reached the gazebo and peed on it. Moo Goo, the eager bride, strained on the leash to reach her groom. The respective parents lifted the couple to a table, and the ceremony began.

Uncle Mort officiated with the solemnity of a priest or rabbi, reading the marriage contract. Dee and her husband gave the bride away. The bride and groom seemed more interested in each other's butt than the service, much to the embarrassment of their owners who had to encourage them a few dozen times to face each other. But Uncle Mort finally pronounced the chows stud and bitch, and the guests applauded, whistled or barked. The bride and groom exchanged a few more sniffs and licks, and then it was time for the guests to eat. Woofer and Moo Goo were excused as they were hot to trot and wanted to consummate their marriage immediately on the table but settled for the privacy of the garage. "Hell, what's the fuss?" said Woofer's father, "They're married."

All the dogs ran for bowls of food placed on the grass and the people headed for tables laden with a catered feast. It was quite a do.

We guests later received thank you notes, complete with a photograph of the bride and groom, signed with their paw prints. They "wrote" that Woofer was very turned on by the gift my wife and I gave, a Fredrick's of Doggywood sheer nightgown. Dee said she was happy that it wasn't the ninth set of matching leads and collars, the fifth bag of rawhide twists or the fourth chew toy shaped like a diamond ring. "It reminds me of the multiple toasters and picture frames Stan and I got as presents."

I have attended several dog weddings over the years. Some simple affairs with only "family" and intimate friends took place in the stud's living room or my clinic; others were more elaborate with 100 or more guests on the lawn of a country club or fine hotel. However, no matter where the weddings took place, regardless of the planning or spontaneity, "parents" and guests had fun and all were affairs to remember.

Any celebration is an affair to remember. Guests who aren't Dog-Gone Owners might have a bit of trouble identifying with what's going on but they sure as hell won't forget the day, or the spirit of fun that prevailed.

Puppy showers were rare, compared to holiday, birthday and wedding parties. And usually there was a darned good reason for having them.

In one case, a childless couple felt left out. Over the years Lisa and her husband had given very nice presents to friends and co-workers who became parents or had more children.

Yet when they bought another beagle and sent out birth announcements, she was upset that most of their friends ignored the significance of the big event. "They knew our beagle is our baby," Lisa told me. Only two friends took the time to respond with congratulatory cards and only one presented the baby with a gift, a fuzzy bear.

"It's not that we need money or gifts, even though having a dog is expensive. We just want our friends to acknowledge that our dogs are as important to us as their children are to them. They're our sons."

Soon after they bought their third dog, Lisa sent puppy shower invitations. "We wanted friends and family to share our joy, to make a little fuss, to bring a gift no matter how piddling. We wanted the same attention that other parents receive. And, we got it!"

Sending the invitations made the people think. Would anyone have three dogs if they didn't love them? Would they celebrate the latest arrival if they weren't serious about welcoming him into their world and their social circle? Would they send invitations for a Sunday afternoon when they knew people generally were free? Would they go to all that trouble for nothing? No way.

If the written word didn't make an impression, seeing one dog sitting in a high-chair where he ate his lunch, the second sleeping in a crib and the baby cavorting in the playpen did. "Now our three dogs get birthday cards and gifts."

While this couple wanted to receive, Ellie and Bob thought it was better to give. Mopsy, their collie, got loose and managed to have a romantic interlude with a dachshund. "How they managed to connect defies gravity and nature considering the difference in their sizes, but connect they did."

When Mopsy delivered six pups, the proud "grandparents" had a baby shower. More accurately, they had a "pick out your pet party."

"We didn't know how else to unload six mixed puppies. People who know Mopsy's so sweet and gentle often said they'd take one of her babies, but they figured we'd breed her with another collie." The baby shower gave their friends the opportunity to stop talking and start taking. Hopefully they'd make dibs on a pup with questionable lineage and "God knows whose looks," and Andrea and Tom could keep the babes within their group.

To a dog lover nothing is as cute as a newborn puppy, and the younger and more helpless it is the more people tend to "ooh and aah." Ellie and Bob briefly considered inviting guests to witness the miracle of birth, but figured some people were bound to be squeamish, and that would defeat the purpose. So, they set the scene for three days later.

When friends arrived at the party, they saw Mopsy in a soft-sided playpen, dressed in a bonnet with a pair of glasses stuck on her nose. Her owners had placed diapers, receiving blankets and various parenting and baby name books around her. "Watching her serenely nurse and clean her tiny puppies made everyone turn into soft mush," Andrea said. "We found good homes for every one. Of course, we had to invite a heck of a lot of people, figuring that a few would be hold outs and nix the idea."

To guarantee that nobody would renege once they said they'd adopt, the grandparents presented the adoptive parents with certificates, a box of dog treats, a collar and leash, and a standing invitation to visit whenever they wished until the babies were weaned and ready to go home with them. "We counted on the parent-child bond and hoped they'd bond like cement. They did," she said with a huge smile.

Many of the happy occasions and parties I attended revolved around religious events.

Butch's christening was celebrated at home with Perrier "holy water." He was dressed in the white gown his human sister had worn to her christening three years before. While some guests could not understand "why, in a zillion years anyone would have an out-in-space party like this," Butch's parents were moved by the service to the point where Mom cried and Dad had tears in his eyes. "Now we're a real family, with a daughter and a son," Mom said, cuddling the baby.

Matilda was spayed before she entered into a life of celibacy and spirituality in the nunnery of her own home. "That's a wonderful reason to celebrate and thank God," her parents said. "We won't have to worry about her being led off the righteous path. We gave her a gold cross to wear on her collar, and that will remind her that there are better things in life than sex." Since that comment came from people who were expecting their seventh child, it took a while for it to compute.

One unforgettable "religious" happy event was Bubba's Bark Mitzvah. His owners somehow figured that their teacup poodle was the equivalent of 13 years of age when he reached 13 months. They knew he wasn't eligible for a real Bar Mitzvah, where a 13 year old boy is considered a man, ready and capable of assuming his religious duty and responsibility. But they could guarantee that their five pound dog would experience a similar ritual. "Bubba's a Jewish dog. He's entitled to the ceremony and the party."

As Bubba tried to paw off the crocheted skullcap tied under his chin, his master addressed the guests. "I'm sorry to say that it has been many years since I attended a Bar Mitzvah, and I've never been to a Bark Mitzvah. Since I don't know what the hell I'm doing but my wife is making me do something, I'm gonna instruct Bubba on my version of the Ten Commandments for dogs." He invited ultra religious people to leave the room. Nobody moved. He then instructed Bubba to bark his affirmation after each sentence. "Understand?" Bubba yipped.

"Very good. Let's continue. I, Bubba shall honor my master and mistress." Not a peek came out of the dog. "That's us, Bubba, Pa and Ma."

"Yip."

"I, Bubba, shall not covet my neighbor's dog, specifically Shana, that sexy bitch next door." No reply from Bubba. His master glared at him, and muttered, "Answer, or no steak tonight."

"Yip."

He, Bubba, agreed not to kill any more of his stuffed animals, steal food off anyone's plate, hump the leg of girls or women who excited him, lie and tell Pa he hadn't had a treat when he had, tattle to Ma when Pa sneaked a smoke, nip his veterinarian when he got injections, or wake Ma or Pa before the sun rose on Sabbath mornings.

Bubba yipped his little heart out. Pa told the standing joke of the Bar Mitzvah boy who thanks his mother and his father, and says, 'Today I am a fountain pen,' because so many guests gave him pens as presents. "Now, Bubba, kiss kiss Ma and kiss kiss Pa." Bubba licked both of them. "In conclusion," Pa said, to the relief of several "congregants" witnessing this momentous occasion, "today you, Bubba, are a . . . ?"

Bubba grabbed a rawhide chew stick out of Pa's pocket, and flipped it in the air. "Right!" Pa said. "I now pronounce you a Bark Mitzvah!"

Everyone in the room shouted, "Mazel Tov!" or "Good luck!" except for one woman who said, "That little runt made such a racket. I'm glad it's over. I was ready to shoot him and his owners."

Bubba had his first taste of wine to celebrate the great occasion and then left the partying to people. Ma claimed it was the best party she and Pa had ever thrown. "Partially because it didn't matter if it didn't go off perfectly. After all, I expected Pa to make mistakes. But the best was that everyone joined in the fun. It would have been nice, though," she said after a small hesitation, "if I didn't have to find a place to stash a lifetime supply of rawhide chews."

Dog parties for any occasion. They're far out, zany, and definitely not an everyday occurrence. It's a shame they're not.

I think Dog-Gone Owners have something that the rest of us miss. We don't celebrate our happy and important times as often as they highlight their pets' milestones, big or small. Maybe we can learn from them that it's good to let down our hair, and do what we want no matter what others think.

And, the more I think about it, the more I think it's a fine idea to belatedly celebrate my Maisie's birthday and try to make up for the times I ignored her day. You're invited to the party.

RSVP regrets only, and no chew-sticks please.

Chapter 9

Dog-Gone Divorces

I'm still honeymooning with my bride of 49 years so divorce hasn't hit me personally. But I've heard enough about the subject from clients to place me one rung below attorneys.

I don't think couples consciously intend to drag me into their divorces but I am a witness to them anyway. Maybe the privacy of the examination room encourages them to confide in me, or the table vaguely reminds them of a psychiatrist's couch. Or maybe, just being confined in a small room with the spouse they are intending to divorce causes them to go over the edge.

All I can say is that whenever a Dog-Gone client mentioned the dreaded "D" word, I reacted with some "D" words of my own—Dismay and Discomfort. I knew from the past that however determined a couple was to maintain a degree of decency through their marital dissolution, it was only a matter of time until one or both sank to a dismal depth of detestable demeanor.

The Goodfriends are a good example. They seemed to be an ideal duo. More than once I told my wife they had that special spark few couples retain after decades of marriage. They were lovers who still flirted with each other, patted each other's fanny and hugged frequently. Unlike one couple I named the "Bickersons," they didn't introduce themselves to the clinic receptionist as "Mrs. Goodfriend and Stupid," or "Mr. Goodfriend and his pain in the ass."

"The Goodfriends will stay married," I told my wife, after one of their lovey dovey visits. "They'll never detonate the 'D' bomb."

"Never say never," she said, raising her eyebrows.

Months later I greeted the smiling couple and their dog, Tootsie, and the first words out of Mr. Goodfriend's smiling mouth were, "We're getting a divorce." I said I was shocked. Missus held her husband's hand in both of hers and told me not to be upset. They both wanted the divorce. They weren't going to be like most other divorcing couples. "We're going to live up to our name and remain good friends. Right, sweetheart?"

"Right, darling. We still love each other," said Mister lifting Tootsie to the table. "We just can't live with each other."

As I began to examine Tootsie, Mrs. Goodfriend anxiously asked me to check the dog's ears. "She keeps pawing at them and whining."

"Will do," I answered.

"Sweetheart," she said to her husband, "I told you we should have brought Tootsie in three days ago when I first noticed she had problems."

"Did you, darling?" he answered. "I didn't hear you."

"Well, sweetie, that's not unusual. You never listen to me."

"Never, love? It seems I've listened to you for 30 years. I've pulled my hair out just listening to you blab about one stupid thing after another."

"Well, honey, that explains why you're bald. I'm happy that you finally revealed some honest feelings. So, I blab about stupid things . . . like our baby's health."

"Control yourself, Toots," he said quite forcibly. "Dr. Vine doesn't need to hear the ravings of an over-emotional female!"

"Hear this, Cue Ball," she boomed, "if I'm over-emotional, you're a zombie! One of the walking dead! I can't wait to get you out of my life!"

By this time Tootsie was whining and had shoved her head into my armpit. "Her ear problem is you," I told the Goodfriends. "She can't stand to hear you yell at each other." Then, they ran out of breath and insults so they tabled their argument, and the remainder of the dog's examination was routine.

This spat is only a sample of divorce-related dialogue I have heard over the years, give or take a few adjectives and nouns. It was just another unpleasant incident where the room temperature plunged from warm to frigid faster than I could take the dog's temperature. And another instance when I waved away curious staff members who were jockeying for position trying to see the battling duo through the small window in the door.

Without doubt divorce transforms some nice, loving, generous people into raving antagonists. I've seen smiles turn to frowns, and heard harmless conversation and polite words give way to snarls and growls. As the arguing intensified, it always amused me that the couple was so intent on verbally murdering each other in the examination room they ignored me. It was as if I had suddenly became invisible, didn't exist.

When I tried to intervene in the early years, I'd hear, "Just a minute, Dr. Vine," before they continued their attack. When I raised my voice, I'd see two heads jerk my way and four eyes stab me, and hear both of them impatiently bark, "WHAT?"

In time I learned to control the situation by throwing my hands in the air, and saying, "Look, I know you people are having troubles, but this isn't the place to air them. Would you prefer we continue Snuffy's exam now? Or should we reschedule it for a time when you intelligent people can be civil to one another?" This usually succeeded in hushing them up long enough for me to do my job, and for my eavesdropping staff to get back to their tasks.

One evening at a cocktail party a lawyer friend noticed I was upset. I had reason to be. Just a few hours before, an irate Dog-Gone Owner had whipped her husband with Tommy Terrier's leash.

"You didn't think I'd find out about your girlfriend?" she had hissed, smacking his knee. "You no good piece of garbage!" Smack, smack. "I'm getting a divorce!" She hit him a few more times. "Custody of Tommy, too!"

It was an amazing scene. By the time she got in her last whack, the gentleman was cowering behind me, pleading, "Lovey, don't hurt Dr. Vine!"

Now I couldn't get into the particulars of these clients with the attorney, but I managed to tactfully steer the conversation to divorce.

"There are three sides to every one," he said. "His, hers and the truth."

"Not so," said a recent divorcee. "There are two sides. Mine and the lying bastard's."

Regardless of the numbers, a tremendous amount of unpleasantness takes place between a couple before divorce attorneys collect their fees. I'm not talking about custody of children, distribution of assets or who gets to keep Aunt Matilda's wedding gift. These decisions are a snap compared to deciding the future of the family dog.

You'd think that if a dog were blessed with one average owner and one Dog-Gone Owner, he'd automatically end up living with the Dog-Gone Owner who desperately wanted him. This could happen when the average owner doesn't want any "left overs" from the spouse hanging around, including the dog.

But average owners have been known to use the dog to emotionally blackmail the Dog-Gone Owner. "You can have the dog if I get everything I want. Hear me? Everything. If not . . ." Then too, some average owners used the dog as a weapon of torture.

One gentleman told me, "It's pay back time." He was fighting for custody of Max. He don't really want him. He hated walking him, loathed the mess he made when he ate and detested his barking.

"I'm going to annoy the crap out of Lucinda. She thinks the sun rises and sets on Max. It's Max this and Max that, and I'm Maxed out of my head. So I'm gonna do a little Maxing of my own. When I think Lucinda is ready to break, I'll magnanimously give in and let her have the damned dog."

This man deliberately punished his wife because he felt she had it coming. "It was bad enough playing second banana to a dog," he told me with tears in his eyes. "But the final straw was when she threw a piece of my life in the dumpster. My high school football letter," he sobbed.

He lived up to his word and gave Lucinda full custody of the dog.

Grinning, he said, "I pushed her far enough. She was ready to go to a psychiatrist, and I didn't want to pay extra alimony to cover those bills."

Being "Maxed out," or resenting taking second place to the family dog, was a complaint that rang a familiar bell throughout my practice. It wasn't necessarily the reason a couple divorced, but it certainly seemed a strong contributing factor.

One divorcee told me, "It's totally demoralizing to be upstaged and replaced by a dog. In my own home, too. I could have fought another woman but how do you fight a dog? Tell her to stop calling? Demand she leave my husband alone or stop sleeping with him? How can I deal with a husband whose priority system is so insane that the dog comes before a wife of 20 years who worked her tail off while the brain went to med school? To hell with marriage . . . and them."

In one case, a husband had surgery and spent months recuperating at home. Bill whiled away the hours feeding Roscoe the Great Dane, walking him, taking naps with him, teaching him tricks (but not good manners), and doting on him.

At first, wife Bobbi didn't object since she worked full time and the puppy was her husband's sole and constant buddy. But on weekends, Roscoe still came first. Bobbi was expected to ignore his jumping on the furniture and raiding food from their plates. When she reprimanded Roscoe, Bill scolded, "He's just a puppy. Leave him alone."

"Several things made my blood boil," Bobbi said. "Bill made bacon and eggs every morning. For Roscoe. He broiled meat and poultry for Roscoe's dinner and fed it to him bit by bit. He stopped taking showers with me and started taking them with Roscoe. In bed, Roscoe slept between us. When we went in the car, Roscoe sat in front with Bill, and I sat in the back seat."

The situation intensified until the couple lost friends. "Because of Bill's obsession with Roscoe," Bobbi said.

They had a terrific fight when Bill insisted on bringing Roscoe to a wedding reception even though the bride's mother, Bobbi's close friend, had called to tell him pets were not invited.

"I asked him to stay home with the dog," Bobbi said. "He refused. He was sure every pet owner would understand. Well, they didn't. The bride's mother had a fit just seeing them. She told Bill that if she had wanted dogs at her daughter's wedding, her Chow would have been the flower girl. Bill got uppity and said, 'If you want Roscoe to leave, just tell me. We'll be happy to go.' She told him to take his dog home. He grabbed my hand. 'If Roscoe isn't welcome, neither are we,' he said, and pulled me to the car. I can't tell you how embarrassed I was. Despite my apologizing many times, our friendship is kaput."

Even after this Bobbi still tried to make the marriage work. She suggested marital counseling. Bill declined, saying there was nothing wrong with him. She was the one with the big problem of jealousy. The crisis came to a head when they were invited to spend a weekend out of state with one of her long time girl friends.

"I told Bill he couldn't bring Roscoe because B.J. had cats and it wasn't fair that she or her pets had to put up with Roscoe. I went alone. An hour later, he drove up with the dog. He had the gall to walk into B.J.'s kitchen and take a turkey she was roasting out of the oven so he could broil a steak he had brought for Roscoe's dinner. That's when B.J. exploded and threw Bill and the dog out, and I started screaming divorce. Now I'm sorry I waited so long. I hope Bill and Roscoe will be very happy together. They deserve each other."

But what happens when both dog owners want custody of the same pet? I'll start with the worst story.

I was fresh out of veterinary school when a couple came to my clinic and requested I put their six month old dachshund to sleep. The dog was in good health, so I asked why they wanted him destroyed. There was no need, I told them, as I could find a good home for such a cute puppy.

"Just do it. Now," said the wife.

Because I was young and inexperienced, I injected a lethal dose into the dog's vein. I'll regret it for the rest of my life.

As soon as the puppy lost consciousness the man and woman became hysterical. Sobbing, they each held the dead dog, and kissed him goodbye. I stood there, watching them, becoming more furious by the minute. If they loved the puppy that much, why had they wanted him dead?

The man explained between sobs that he and his wife were getting divorced. They both loved the dog dearly but they couldn't bear to see the other person or any person get him. They decided no one would have him.

That was a first and last for me. From then on, whenever any divorcing Dog-Gone Owners asked me to perform euthanasia on their healthy pets I told them to find another vet. Maybe they did. I don't know as I never saw these clients again. I like to think I shamed them into changing their minds.

On a lighter note is the couple that divorced and then remarried; not because they loved each other, but because they loved Patsy the bulldog. After the dissolution, Ma got custody of the dog and the house, and Pa got unlimited visitation rights that he abused from day one. He'd drop by before breakfast to see Patsy, spend the day in his easy chair with his feet on the ottoman and the dog in his lap, and remain until he read her a bed time story. (See illustration 28)

"He became a habit, again," said Ma, "when he started sleeping in his bedroom." This time around Ma made ground rules. They had to remarry so Patsy wouldn't reside with two

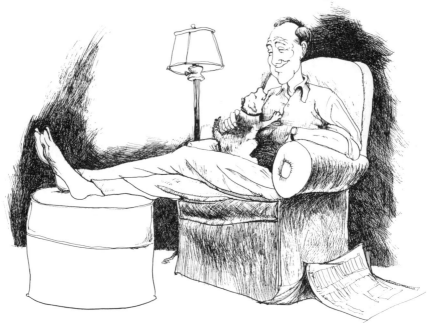

28. Helping people relax

sinful people. They were to allow Patsy to decide which person she wanted to sleep with, instead of fighting over her. And, if Patsy ended up snuggled next to Ma, Pa was not to tiptoe into Ma's bedroom in the dead of night, abduct the dog and sneak her into his room. "The first time he breaks the rules, we get divorced again." Since they stayed together until Pa died, I assume he reformed.

When we speak of divorce and dog custody, we usually think of husband versus wife. There was an instance though, that involved parents versus their child when the daughter moved out of her parents' home, taking along Hogan, a mixed terrier.

"She hurt us terribly when she moved into her own apartment and ripped away our son," said Mom. "We want Hogan back. He's our dog, not hers!" they insisted, "and we won't give him up!"

They asked their daughter to return the pet. They pleaded with her. She wouldn't budge.

One day they called and asked to visit Hogan, and the daughter reluctantly agreed. The parents gave Hogan some new toys and treats, played with him, fussed over him, hugged and kissed him. Then the mother asked her daughter to make a pot of coffee. While she was in the kitchen, they dognapped Hogan.

"They were out the door in a split second," the daughter told me. "When I got to their house, their car was in the garage. I banged on the door. They wouldn't let me in. I tried using my keys. They wouldn't work because they had changed the locks. This was premeditated! My own parents did this to me, their only child!" she cried.

Things went from bad to worse. Mom and Dad refused to let their daughter visit Hogan. She threatened to sue them. They threatened to boycott her wedding, and did. She retaliated by taking them to court. At the trial, the judge ordered dual custody of the dog, and suggested, "The affection lavished on this dog would be better lavished on each other."

"What an idiot thing for a judge to say. He doesn't know my dog or my daughter. He's lucky I didn't punch him in the nose," said Dad. (See illustration 29.)

I thought the judge was wise ordering dual custody as a means of appeasing all the parties. But I guess his decision was similar to looking at a glass and being happy that it's half full while someone else sees it as half empty. Hogan's family all felt cheated.

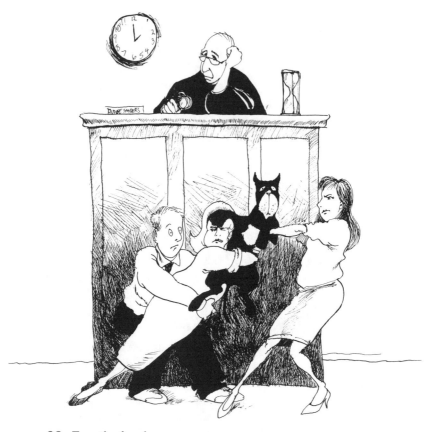

29. Family feud

The mother told me, "I don't like having to give him up every other week, but it's better than out and out warfare."

However, the daughter reported, "I'll never be able to forgive the judge. And I'll never trust my parents from now on. Whenever they have Hogan I expect them to dog-nap him again so they don't ever have to give him back to me."

So much for blood being thicker than water.

A surprising number of divorces have to be resolved in the courtroom solely because of the family dog. The German philosopher, Friedrich Nietzsche, once said, "In revenge and in love woman is more barbarous than man." Evidently Nietzsche hadn't talked to divorced dog owners. If he had, he would have given the sexes equal credit, and the divorce judge a bottle of tranquilizers.

It can't be easy for any sympathetic judge who likes animals to decide the fate of a pet. Not with two rabid Dog-Gone Owners battling over the family pooch.

According to law, a dog is considered personal property. According to opinionated owners, the state law is preposterous. How can a judge plunk a dog in the same basket as a salt shaker, Rolls Royce, gold or diamonds? We're talking about a living and breathing, one-of-a-kind, irreplaceable treasure that is sometimes more precious than children. And as sure as God makes fleas, Dog-Gone Owners will fight each other with fangs and claws to gain 100% custody of their pet. This is especially true when there are no children in the family.

Sweetie Pie was the world to his childless owners, Jean and Roy, who divorced after a four-year marriage. The judge decreed the dog a "child substitute" and ordered the couple to share her on alternate months. That worked well until Sweetie Pie ran away from home and had a romantic interlude with an amorous poodle who, in the vernacular, knocked her up.

The couple went back to court.

"She should be with her mother at a time like this," Jean told the judge.

"What does she know about mothering?" Roy said. "I'll up my offer of $35,000 to $50,000 and throw in my life-sized portrait of Sweetie Pie if she'll give me permanent and sole custody."

"Take your filthy money and keep the portrait. Sweetie Pie's pregnant and she needs me!"

Alas, the judge didn't agree. He ruled that the dog was to continue spending alternating months with the couple and the portrait was to be loaned to Jean whenever Roy had the expectant mother. "And both of you will be with the dog when she's delivering her puppies, no matter who she's with that month." He also instructed them to keep and share, on the months they didn't have Sweetie Pie, one pup from the litter. "That should help salve the lonesome blues," he said, banging his gavel. "Case dismissed."

The couple was appeased but not elated. When it comes to possessive owners, it's a case of all or nothing at all, and the all should come to me. Only cloning the dog so each ex-spouse could have full custody would make them happy.

Various divorced Dog-Gone clients told me that sharing their dog with their ex was actually harder than not having custody at all. "It's sort of like my child died," one woman explained "But if that were the case, I'd know I'd never see him again. Instead, every year I have to say goodbye to my baby for six months. No visitation or contact because my ex lives 2000 miles away. So every year I go into mourning, have to get used to an empty house and adjust to being alone. It's terribly depressing until the baby is back in my home. Then for six months I feel like I'm reborn, only to go through the separation again."

Another divorcee said, "Shared custody stinks. Because of Flippy, my ex put me through hell. I really hate him but we'll always be connected through the dog. Give up Flippy? Never. I want my ex to suffer like I do."

I asked if she thought another puppy would help ease her pain. She said it probably would, but she feared Flippy would experience sibling rivalry. "I couldn't risk that."

But, talk to those who lost custody, and they think alternating months or six consecutive months is better than winning the lottery.

"They're very lucky. I lost custody," one man told me. "It's agonizing. I call every day to find out how the dog is and my ex answers the phone. She tells me to shove off, to stop calling and bothering her. Do you think I like speaking to her? She made my life miserable for 14 years. Then, to make things worse, I had to hand over the one person who means more to me than anyone else on earth. My poodle, Cookie." Then he whispered, "I'm planning to dog-nap her."

Several divorced clients mentioned dog-napping. Most of these people believed it was the dirtiest and most inexcusable but well deserved trick one divorced Dog-Gone Owner could pull on another. But it's not often carried out because of the deterrents.

It means life on the run, a gypsy existence for people who previously enjoyed having their roots firmly planted in familiar territory. It entails giving up a job and benefits and finding another way to support yourself and your dog. It's looking over your shoulder to make sure your ex hasn't found you. "It's awful. I feel like a fugitive," a dog-napper told me, "and I guess I am."

One ex-husband told me he had been awarded full custody of his dog. "I am the better parent, you know," he gloated. His wife had visitation rights, "one over-nighter a week and every Sunday." The arrangement went smoothly until one Sunday evening when his ex had not returned the dog at the specified time. He drove to her apartment to discover she had moved. She had left no forwarding address. Her phone was disconnected. No new number. The next day he went to her work place. She had quit the previous Friday. He called her parents. They hadn't heard from their daughter. He spoke to some of her neighbors and every friend he could find. Nobody could or would help him. "I was in shock. I knew my ex was devious but I couldn't believe she'd do that to me."

The next day instead of going to work he went to a detective agency with photos of his ex and his dog. "I'll pay anything to get him back."

Several weeks later, the detective called to say he had located the woman in Arizona, and he had seen the dog.

The owner took the next plane to Scottsdale, rented a car, and parked it across the street from the house where his ex lived. "I got there a few minutes before Sport's dinner time because I knew she'd let him out to do his business as soon as he was through eating." The man wasn't disappointed. The apartment door opened, his ex stood in the doorway and Sport bounced out to the lawn. "It was the perfect chance!"

Did he get his dog back? No.

The gentleman was so happy to see his dog he became paralyzed. He couldn't call him, couldn't move or jump out of the car to snatch him. His ex spotted him sitting in the car, and whistled for Sport who ran back inside. As the man sat there crying and pounding the steering wheel because he had missed his opportunity, his ex sneaked out the back door with suitcases and drove off with the dog. As of today, thousands of dollars later, there's still no clue where they are.

Now the gentleman is in therapy, trying to pull himself together and heal the ulcers and insomnia that plague him. "Depressed doesn't even come close to describing the way I feel. I want to kill myself. If I can't get Sport back, life isn't worth living."

From what he said, his family and friends have not been very supportive, but then they're not Dog-Gone Owners. "They don't understand. They just tell me to get another dog. As if I could ever replace Sport. He's my child, my son."

One victim of dog-napping said, "Having my ex-husband do this to me is like having an enemy steal the child you conceived, carried, delivered and reared. Not a day goes by that I don't think about Bosco, worry about him and wish my ex was six feet under."

Giving them the benefit of the doubt, let's say that most obsessed dog owners are unable to recognize that their priority system is a bit unusual.

Ironically, though, if both husband and wife consider the dog before each other, blindly love and dote on the pet, they're in accord about one issue even if their marriage is falling apart. Sometimes that's enough to keep them together. So what if you're married to a person who treats you like a dog and treats the dog like a person? That's nothing compared to disrupting a dog's life. One husband said, "How can I divorce the woman? Jocko is innocent and helpless. He needs both of us to love him."

Yet, when you least expect it, a divorcing Dog-Gone Owner will do the admirable thing, like placing her children ahead of her dogs.

Isabella believed her four terriers and not her two children needed her love and attention. The kids let her know they resented the fuss she made over the pets. Her young son complained to me that he didn't have a middle name but all of the dogs did . . . Remy Martin Saldano, Jack Daniel Saldano, Rob Roy Saldano and Tia Maria Saldano. "And she bakes cookies for the dogs but buys us yucky stuff at the store. And one year she was so busy making a birthday party for one of the dogs, she forgot my sister's birthday."

To say this woman was gaga over her dogs is putting it mildly. Yet, when she and her husband divorced, and both wanted the terriers, she surprised everyone by keeping the children and giving her ex full custody of the dogs. This generated a lot of gossip, and people speculated why she had made such an unexpected decision. One friend claimed, "She knows she can't get child support for the kids and the dogs, and she will get more for the kids than the dogs. Ergo, kids."

But one charitable soul told me, "I think she had a spiritual experience."

"Like what?" I asked.

"Oh, I don't know. Maybe she finally realized that real people don't have tails and fur."

Most enthralled owners recognize the needs of their children exceed those of their pets. And as crazy as they are about their dogs, they manage to be good parents, too. But every now and then a Mom and a Dad don't agree on priorities, and there's trouble in paradise.

One of my clients called her husband "Mr. Perfect" in their early years of marriage. Jacob was the perfect husband. They had a perfect daughter. Life was perfect. Then they got two Maltese puppies. Life and Jacob changed.

"We're getting a divorce," she told me during a visit.

"Yippee," he said, "I can't wait."

Evidently, when Jacob came home from work he kissed the dogs before he kissed his wife and daughter. "I've tried giving him puppy dog eyes," Dina said, glaring at Jacob. "He ignored me. Our three-year-old daughter tried crawling to him on all fours and yipping for attention like the dogs. He ignored her, too. He finally admitted the dogs were the most important to him, then me; our little girl came last."

He interrupted her to say, "But you were a close second."

"If the house caught on fire, Dr. Vine, he'd save the dogs first," Dina said.

"Of course I would," he answered. "Why are you upset?"

"You don't know why I'm upset?" she cried. "Listen to your words!"

"Hey, when I get home from work, I want a little attention. The dogs are always there but your head is in the oven, checking the roast."

"The roast is for you. Remember?" she said, shaking her head in disgust. "What about our daughter? You don't spend time with her, either. You take the dogs for walks. Why can't you take her along?"

"She's too much trouble," he said, in my presence.

Another wife complained to me about her non-existent love life. "Well, maybe you should try harder," her husband told her.

"When it's three against one? The dogs and you on one side of the bed, and me on the other? You don't let our son in bed with us after he has a nightmare, but the dogs sleep with us every night. The last time I asked you to put them on the floor, you almost bit my head off."

"Well, I love them," he said.

"So do I! But not as much as our son," she said. "Dr. Vine, he told me if I left and took our boy that would be all right. But if I took one of the dogs he'd hunt me down and hurt me."

"I also said if she took both dogs, I'd kill her," he added. I believed him.

Another divorcing couple debated one issue after another for two years. Finally, child custody was established, the property settlement was resolved and alimony was determined. All that was left to fight over was Tuffy, a sweet but very ugly dog.

Dominic said, "Angelica can have the children. I want Tuffy." Claiming that it would be harmful for the dog to be shifted back and forth between his home and Angelica's, he filed for full custody, and won. As an attorney he had the know-how, contacts, and money to get his way. "It was worth every cent," he said.

Sadly, few divorce stories involving Dog-Gone Owners have happy endings for both parties. Even when they end up with the dog, even with a new love interest, some folks seemed incapable of putting the experience behind them. They get a perverse pleasure holding on to their hatred of their ex.

One divorcee told me, "I'm gonna make the SOB suffer for the rest of his life for what he did to me." Her way to make him suffer was to call him in the middle of the night every year on their divorce anniversary, bark and howl, and yell, "Gotcha!" before she slammed down the receiver. This continued for seven years. The next year he beat her at her own game. "It wasn't fun any more, so I stopped," she told me. "No, that's not true. I did it once more, told him I hoped he'd burn in hell, and then stopped."

I've had married clients who have divorced, married others and had two or three children with their second mates. But because they didn't get full custody of the dog, or they were unhappy about sharing custody or they hated the visitation arrangements, they still dreamed of terminating their previous mates.

Two women were talking about this when one said she would love to plunge a knife into her ex and twist it. "If I were to actually do something," the second one said, "I'd choose a carving fork. Stab and twist. Does more damage."

Another client dashed into my clinic, threw her arms up in the air, shook her hips, and yelled, "Hallelujah! I'm free! I'm free! Thank God, I'm free!" For a minute I was afraid some of the clients in the reception area might have thought they were in a faith healer's temple. By the time I ran over to her, the clients were staring at her as if she were mad, their dogs were barking and their cats were meowing.

"What are you talking about?" I whispered, hastily ushering her into an examination room. "You've been single for years."

"Right. Five years. But my ex dropped dead! Now I start to live again! I finally get the dog!"

Well, we know that Dog-Gone Owners often choose pets over people, especially people they want to hurt. But I often felt that fighting over the family pet was a smoke screen that kept a couple from acknowledging major problems that had existed in the marriage for a long time.

One little corgi, Beauty, started to have epileptic fits. Of course her owners rushed her to the clinic, but I couldn't find a thing wrong with her. Then she had another seizure, and another. Now, each time I saw Beauty, I asked the owners, "Is anything going on at home? Any problems?" They always claimed everything was fine.

Finally, Beauty had a seizure and the couple put the puzzle pieces together. When they fought it was always over the dog, even though they admittedly were angry for other reasons. But instead of confronting the big issues, they went haywire over trivial things, such as how much to feed their pet, how long to walk her, or how often to have her groomed.

Since her owners were on the verge of divorce and both had volatile tempers, their fights were becoming increasingly violent.

"She throws dishes at me," he said, pointing the finger at his wife.

"He screams at me and pounds holes in the walls!" she countered.

"She hits me."

"He hits back."

I advised them to settle their differences . . . "if that's possible" . . . elsewhere. "Your Beauty, like all dogs, is completely aware of your emotional ups and downs. She's reacting to them. They're triggering her epileptic seizures. In other words, you're the cause. I don't care how much you two hate each other, if you love your dog, you'll spare her."

Reluctantly they decided to try marital counseling to see if that would help. It took 18 months, "and some of those months were absolutely horrendous," the wife said, but they resolved enough of their long-standing problems to realize they still loved each other and wanted to stay together. As the tension lessened, Beauty's epilepsy tapered off, reappearing only briefly when she became a big sister to a real baby girl.

At the other end of the spectrum were married clients who swore they had never fought nor had disagreements throughout their union. This is incomprehensible to me since I believe in clearing the air and making up, even if it necessitates putting cotton in the dog's ears to protect her from loud discussions.

I interpreted total and constant harmony to mean that one of the spouses was devoid of hearing, speech and sight; although it was clear both had full use of their senses. Well then, I thought, maybe one spouse was born without any buttons to push, so the other person stopped trying to find them. However, since World War III had broken out during the divorce, this wasn't the case either. Apparently every ugly retort the couple repressed and every disagreeable thought they hadn't communicated during the marriage years was remembered, mentally listed and counted, and expressed in the dog fights.

Consider Quincy and Gert.

If asked to describe them, I'd say she was a combination Joan Rivers and Leona Helmsley, a non-stop talker and assertive woman. Quincy was Casper Milquetoast, quiet and henpecked. Whatever she said, he'd answer, "Yes, dear." Whatever he whispered, she'd reply, "Quincy, hush up, I'm talking."

Then, much to the surprise of Gert, Quincy filed for divorce. "He never said one harsh word to me in 32 years," Gert said, "and the word divorce never crossed his lips until now." I decided that was because Quincy never had the chance to get in a word in sideways.

Next I heard, "Quincy is fighting like a bear for Fleasbee. He wants full custody." Then I heard he used Gert's infrequent fainting spells as the reason Fleasbee couldn't be entrusted to her, even for weekly visitation. Finally I heard that immediately after the divorce, Quincy mailed Gert a hefty gift-wrapped package.

"Poop. Fleasbee's poop. It had to be at least three years worth!" Gert said.

But what really astonished her was the accompanying note. "Dear Gert. You gave me nothing but shit for 24 years. Now it's your turn to get some. Love, Quincy."

"You know," Gert said with a sly smile, "this is a new Quincy. I like this guy! I think I'll invite him over for dinner and tell him."

They got back together. You can imagine my delight when Gert led the way into the examination room, and said, "This is the problem with Fleasbee . . .," to which Quincy said, "Gert, sit down and shut up," and she said, "Yes, Dear."

Go figure out Dog-Gone Owners.

One of my favorite divorce stories has a happy ending because the couple fell back in love, and spared their dog from being a product of a permanently broken home.

Roberta and Kenneth battled over Chauncy's custody for almost a year, went to court and were ordered by the judge to share him. "Chauncy was like a child to me," Kenneth said. "When the judge told me I could have my baby only 50% of the week it was like having my son taken away." Roberta told me essentially the same.

Whenever they had to see each other long enough to transfer the dog, they fought bitterly. Meanwhile the dog was going from bad to worse. Chauncy had no appetite, lost weight and hid in closets and under beds.

As Chauncy deteriorated, the arguments got worse, the blame flew back and forth more frequently, and all three became nervous wrecks. Finally the owners called a truce so they could try to help the dog. They took him to an animal psychologist who insisted they'd have to resolve their personal differences for Chauncy's physical and emotional well being.

"That was the last thing we wanted to hear or do," Roberta said. "But we decided to fake it and pretend we were friends again, for Chauncy's sake." The dog reacted favorably. Then Roberta called Ken one day and suggested that maybe it would be less stressful to Chauncy if they arranged his transfer on neutral territory. "Not Ken's apartment or mine. Somewhere public where we couldn't go at each other and yell like lunatics. The post office lawn became the place."

Chauncy began to noticeably improve, so they kept at it. After several months they realized they were able to talk about mundane things and exchange a few laughs. A couple of times they even took Chauncy for short walks before they parted. Then because they were able to stand being with each other without fighting they decided to again try "home deliveries." And, as long as she was at his apartment, or he was at her apartment, they started to make dinners for each other. Then one night there was a terrific rain storm that threatened to put Chapel Hill under water. It was too dangerous for Ken to drive back to his apartment, so he stayed over at Roberta's one-bedroom apartment. "Etcetera, etcetera, etcetera," he said.

Hey, there's more than one way to scratch a dog's fleas.

As far as my staff was concerned, they liked nothing better than happy endings to a divorce story. Dog lovers all, they worried about pets that had to endure life with the Bickersons, dual residency or separation from loved ones. They fumed when they overheard what took place in the homes of sparring couples. The men swore and the women cried when they saw the toll divorce had on some dogs. They even cried when there was a happy ending.

"Have you heard the news?" one of my female staffers sniffled.

"Isabella got Remy Martin, Jack Daniel, Rob Roy and Tia Maria back!"

"That's a surprise," I said.

"And her ex has the kids!"

"That's a shocker. I wonder why."

"Because his new wife is terribly allergic to dog dander and loves children but can't have them. Now everyone's happy. Isn't that wonderful?"

Just another surprising ending to a Dog-Gone divorce.

Chapter 10

That Big Kennel In The Sky

Nancy and I were chitchatting as I examined her bull dog Klutzie when she casually announced, "I've turned into a statistic since I last saw you."

"What do you mean?" I asked.

"My husband died last week. I've joined the ranks of widows."

This wasn't the first time a client told me his or her spouse had died. But never before had a survivor reported the news so calmly. Usually there were heart wrenching sobs, and sometimes the dog joined in, baying and howling with unhappiness. That day Nancy seemed composed, too composed, and old Klutzie seemed his usual self. This discombobulated me.

I knew how to respond to clients who expressed grief. I'd pat their hand or hug them as I said I was sorry. I'd agree that they had lost their only love, "an angel," the best husband or wife that God ever created. Sometimes I cried with people at the time of their loss, too. This time I didn't know what to say to the widow who obviously was in shock and reacting to the traumatic life change by humming "Happy Days Are Here Again."

I reached across the examination table to pat her hand, and gave my usual response. "Nancy, I'm very sorry."

"Don't be," she answered. "We all die. That's life."

That was the last comment I expected to hear from her. I was so shocked that I hid my face in Klutzie's back, and began to laugh from nervousness. Mistaking my laughter for tears, she patted my head and handed me a tissue. "Listen, Dr. Vine, I know you think he was a good man but I don't want you to waste one tear on him. From the day I married him he was a bastard."

Then Klutzie died a few years later, and Nancy's reaction was a little different.

My receptionist told me I had better hurry into the recovery room, a room generally reserved for patients following surgery. Often, however, we escorted nervous owners there before a pet's surgery so they could endure the "endless hours of waiting" in relative peace. Besides magazines and coffee and tea, we occasionally offered the more frantic Dog-Gone Owners a tranquilizer, or gave them first aid if they fainted . . . and several did. Nancy was there with Klutzie's cold body and two friends. "She's a basket case," my receptionist whispered. "I think she's ready to collapse. Let me know when I should call the paramedics."

I entered the small room and saw Nancy sitting in a chair, clutching Klutzie. Her friends appeared upset and completely bewildered as they fanned her face. Nancy looked up at the ceiling, and wailed, "Oh God, why Klutzie?" Moments later,

when God had not answered her question, she looked at me
as if I had the information.

"Nancy, Klutzie was 12 years old. It was his time to die,"
I said.

"I don't care," she cried. "It isn't fair." She held out a hand
and one friend gave her a tissue from the box she was holding.

"Sometimes life isn't fair," I answered, feeling like the king
of cliches. "Remember, you told me that we all die? That
death is part of life?"

"Screw what I said. I didn't mean Klutzie's death."

"But Nancy," the other friend said, "Klutzie was a dog. He
wasn't a husband or child, thank goodness."

"He was better than a husband or child. He was everything
to me," she whispered. "He was my love, my best friend, an
angel, my reason for living. What am I going to do without
him?"

"You'll get over it," the tissue friend said. "I lost my husband less than a year ago. I still miss him terribly, but life
goes on."

"You don't know anything," snarled Nancy. "You've never
lost a dog, a Klutzie. I've been through both. Take it from
me, losing a dog is much worse than losing a mate."

Obviously we weren't getting anywhere. The debate of dog
death versus person death raged on until I said, "Ladies, let's
end this by saying that losing anyone we love is terrible, be it
man or dog. Nancy, why are you here?" She glared at me.
"I mean, as much as I'd like to, there's nothing I can do
for Klutzie."

"Why am I here?" she asked, with an incredulous look on
her face. "I need help arranging his funeral, that's why. I'm
in no condition to do it."

"But you are," I assured her. "Who loved him more and
knew him better than you? Who knows what kind of service
he would have wanted? You. That's who."

"You're right," she agreed, nodding her head and mopping her tears. Then, as one friend flipped her tissues and the other took notes, we discussed funeral arrangements. Nancy went home to plan a send-off for Klutzie that would make him the envy of his friends in that big kennel in the sky.

I knew it would be more elaborate than her husband's, as the tissue lady told me, "She had Waldo cremated. She wanted to flush his ashes down the commode but we convinced her to scatter them. She did, in the city dump."

Most Dog-Gone Owners aren't as biased as Nancy. Yet, the death of a dog can affect them as much or more than the death of a spouse. One client told me she expected her husband to die, and she expected to die. "But somehow, and I know this sounds a little irrational, I don't expect my basset, Bernie, to die. I picture him being around forever. If he goes before we do that will kill us." I understood what she meant.

One of my clients refused to consider that his aging pet would die until he had to face his own death. "I've accepted it," the widower told me. "More than that, I'm getting ready."

I asked him what he meant. "I'll tell you when the time comes," he said.

A couple of months later he called me at home. "I don't want you to be upset by what I'm about to tell you. Promise you won't?"

"I'll try."

He told me that he and his dog planned a double suicide. "Mimi Mutt and I are dying together. I've been socking away some of my morphine pills. I've had enough pain and so has old Mimi. We're going together."

I went into a speech about hospice and pain-free dying, how he shouldn't take things into his hands, how if he loved Mimi he wouldn't kill her. I said everything I could think of saying.

"You don't understand," he told me in a very quiet voice. "We're tired of the physical pain and missing my wife, and we're ready. It's essential that I don't leave Mimi behind. Even for a short time." They talked about it, he said, they agreed, and there was nothing I could do to change their minds. Suddenly I realized he was slurring his words.

"She couldn't live without me, without falling asleep with her head on my chest and feeling me breathing any more than I could live without her, without feeling her softness and seeing the love in her eyes. We've been dying by inches, anyway."

"I'm calling the police."

"Too late," he murmured. "Left town, won't find us, can't find us in time. Bye, Doc." With that he hung up the phone.

Two days later I read in the newspaper that a maid found him and Mimi in a motel bed. Mimi's head was on his chest; his hand was on her back. The suicide note he left explained it all.

Neighbors were shocked to read the news. It was upsetting in itself to know he had killed himself. "But I would have taken the dog, dammit," one dog lover said. "He didn't have to kill her. How could he have been so selfish?"

"Can't you see he found the perfect solution?" another retorted. "They're all together now."

Since it's reality that pets don't last as long as people, death is a matter I often wanted to address with various owners. Generally I didn't have to broach the subject with average clients. They were the ones who brought it up. They would say they knew the dog was aging. "He's slowing down." "She can barely walk." "I can tell he's in pain." "None of the medicines work." "I'm beginning to think about putting her to sleep." "He's going to die soon."

Yet my extreme owners tended to avoid the subject with a passion. This was true even when the pet did everything but shove his snout under the owner's nose to plead, "I know it hurts you to think about my death, but look at me! I'm blind, I'm lame, I'm as old as the hills, and my time's almost here. Don't you think we should start making some plans?" My Dog-Gone Owners did not want to know.

While they could be open about their own end, they refused to talk about the pet's death. They didn't even want to think about it. They'd comment that Poochie looked adorable with missing teeth. Or they joked about taking the dog to the beauty parlor to touch up a graying coat. With clients like these, I kept my mouth shut.

Often I was sorry that I hadn't spoken up. This was especially the case if a client insisted that Poochie was fine and would recover when it was apparent that the dog was very old, terminally ill or terribly injured.

Was it better to try to prepare owners for the inevitable? Or was it kinder to let them continue to fantasize about the wonders of veterinary medicine and the immortality of their pets? To tell or not to tell? I see-sawed back and forth until one day Ollie abruptly settled it.

Ollie was a very old pointer with a bad heart. Despite medications, he was getting worse. His owner, Ruthie, didn't want to face this. Knowing that she was the Queen of Denial, I had decided it would be pointless to point out to Ruthie that her pointer was at death's door. Then, just as I was beginning a routine examination, Ollie passed out.

With my own heart missing a few beats, I checked Ollie's heartbeat. No doubt about it, Ollie was with the angels.

"Ollie just died, Ruthie."

"No, he didn't, Lou. He's cat-napping. He snoozes lots these days. He's lazy, like me."

"Ruthie, he died. He's dead."

"Lou, you're crazy. Wake up, Ollie." Ruthie shook the dog. "Ollie! Wake up! Lou, Ollie won't wake up!" She shook him harder, slapped him, pinched him, and of course Ollie didn't react. If he hadn't been dead, Ruth would have killed him in her berserk attempts to rouse him. She finally looked at me, and screamed, "Murderer! You killed my dog!" I swear I didn't; I had only removed the rectal thermometer.

That experience convinced me that it was wise to discuss the subject of death before the fact. At times it seemed to work. Then again, at times it didn't.

Freda came in with Splotch after he tried to attack a Cadillac head on. The dog was so badly and irreparably injured he was less than one inch away from death.

"He just needs a little fixing up," Freda said.

"Freda, Splotch is not going to make it."

"You're wrong. How's your wife?"

"Fine. But Splotch is in very bad shape. He's suffering. He hurts."

"He's still alive. How are your kids?"

"Great. But Splotch is dying. We should help him die."

"No, he'll be fine."

Mercifully, Splotch took his last breath a moment later. Freda looked at his mangled, bloody body, and asked, "What happened? He just looked a little messed up." She was completely dazed. She talked about having to go outside to walk Splotch. She rambled on incoherently about vacations they were planning to take, buying him a new blanket, and giving him booster shots. Then the realization hit her, she collapsed and we had to call the paramedics.

From then on, I insisted on discussing death even if the client didn't like it, even when it made no impression.

I'd say, "Poochie already lived past his breed's expectancy. Most of his brothers and sisters die long before this. You know, he's slowing down a lot. One of these days . . ."

They'd answer, "You're kidding, Doc. He's in great shape."

"I'm not kidding. Poochie is 12, has arthritis and trouble walking, he's blind, has heart trouble, no teeth and . . . "

"He's just a little under the weather."

All ended up a lot under the weather, like six feet under. Then came the ordeal of facing the death of a loved one.

Both average and Dog-Gone Owners grieved when they lost a pet, and rightfully so. Some stoic clients tried to bottle their emotions by pretending the death was no great loss; but eventually they went through the grieving process anyway. Most, however, reacted immediately and intensely. Some average owners were surprised. "I didn't realize I loved him this much until now," one client cried.

I'd like to have a box of tissues for each man or woman who cried or became hysterical in my clinic. This, to me, was a healthy reaction. Unfortunately, some Dog-Gone Owners prolonged their anguish for months, even years, and it was not unusual for some to become depressed, physically ill, suicidal or alcoholic. Here's a sampling of some clients whose suffering took unusual paths.

Mr. X, one of the nicest clients I had, professed a taste for an "occasional brew" after his pet's death. "It helps to kill the pain," he told me. I guess dropping in to the clinic to say hello helped, too. He began to come in tipsy, and we'd gently usher him to the door. Then a few months later he came in and told me he didn't want to leave. He sat on the reception room floor, took a nip from the bottle he pulled out of his pocket and quietly cried for his dead dog. I called his wife. I think the main reason she made him join AA was that she walked into the clinic just as he made a lunge at an attractive client and invited her to make a puppy with him.

One woman took the death of her poodle so hard that she developed a case of shingles that lasted six months. She finally recovered, she claimed, because her other dog comforted her. "Bif understood how much I hurt both emotionally and physically. He'd put his darling face on my knee and look at me, and say, 'Mom, you have to shape up because I'm still here and I need you.' I knew I had to get better for his sake."

Frank told me he was ready to swallow sleeping pills. "Life without Fuzzy was getting harder and harder to endure. I put up a good front with my friends, acting as if losing Fuzzy was no big deal. I'd change the subject if they wanted to talk about her, and then I'd go home and think about her. All I wanted to do was join her. They didn't know how long and hard I had been thinking about killing myself."

One day, minutes after Frank took out the bottle of sleeping pills and filled the water glass, a friend with cancer visited him. "He said he'd feel better about dying if he knew I'd adopt his dog when he was no longer capable of caring for her. This guy was dying and worried about his dog, and I was healthy but ready to end it all because of my dead dog. That helped me put things in perspective."

Surprising, at least to me, was that the mourners seemed to adjust to their loss faster the more they gave in to it. "It makes me feel much better to cry and carry on whenever I want no matter where I am," a client said, "and I don't give a hang who sees me. I have a hole in my heart."

One gentleman isolated himself for a month. He kept his blinds closed and his doors locked. He, like many other Dog-Gone Owners, said he needed time and solitude to adjust to the shock. "I thought he had killed himself because I called and called and he never picked up the phone," his daughter told me. She finally used her key to let herself into her dad's home, and found him adding photos of Doffo's funeral to a picture album. "It made him feel a little better."

But nothing seems to console a grieving owner more than the beautiful memories of a great send off.

Many is the time I've been a Doctor Kevorkian who helped usher a terminally ill or aged dog into the next life via a painless injection. Once that was over, and if the owner desired, I would dispose of the body. For special clients who requested, "Please, you take care of it," I'd bury dogs in the back of my clinic at no charge. Later, many of these owners erected headstones or markers, and they returned often to visit their departed pets.

Yet, it wasn't at all unusual for clients to leave my clinic and take the dead dog to their house or apartment. There, owners didn't have to make snap decisions about the final resting place for their pet. They could weigh their options in privacy before deciding on a meaningful journey to heaven for the dog.

Katie, a tiny woman, told me she carried her large Doberman to his bed in the kitchen and arranged him so it looked as if he were napping with his paws over his nose, "Like he always did." She talked to him while she prepared his favorite meal of sausage, scrambled eggs and toast, and filled his water bowl with ice-cubes and Perrier. Then she sat on the floor near him while she ate a peanut butter and jelly sandwich. "I knew he was dead, and that he wouldn't eat the food or drink the water, but I had to have one last meal with him before I could bury him in the back yard. Keeping him close was the right thing to do for him and me."

One client invited friends and relatives to Blackie's funeral at a pet cemetery. When I arrived, a friend directed me into the "slumber room" where the mourners were sitting. In front of them, flanked by huge candles and beautiful bouquets of flowers, was the miniature Jewish poodle dressed in a yarmulke (skull cap), tuxedo and bow tie, and laid out in a satin lined casket with a lace pillow.

The casket was a mite crowded for a toy poodle because Blackie's owners wanted him buried with his favorite blanket, squeaky cat toy and a bowl filled with sauteed chicken livers. A chapel employee said a short prayer for Blackie, and his grief stricken owners delivered their eulogy. Then, leading the way for the mourners, Blackie's master carried the casket to the grave site. After the brief ceremony, the casket was lowered into the ground where, following custom in the Jewish religion, each tearful, sad or sheepish looking guest shoveled in a little soil.

While I doubt that Blackie cared what his "parents" did for his send-off, they felt that the $900 casket, $550 funeral, and the $800 tombstone (that would be revealed at the "unveiling" several months later) were worth every penny and then some. Because the family announced they were "sitting shivah," a period of formal mourning following the interment, we went back to Blackie's house to pay further condolences and talk about the dear departed soul while we ate catered food.

Some empathetic guests thought the day was beautiful, and asked Blackie's parents for names and addresses of all the tradespeople, "When the time comes I know where to go to have a beautiful affair for my baby."

"Eternal Tail Waggers is a lovely place, too," one couple offered. They should know. Believers in pre-planning, they had purchased a "companion site" for their four dogs, two still alive and two buried side by side. "We had beautiful services for our dogs when they died. The only thing that saddens us is that Eternal doesn't bury people."

Other folks, though, thought the pet funeral was senseless, and didn't hesitate to voice their opinions. "All this fuss for a poodle? No wonder psychiatrists stay in business." "For Chrissake, we could take a cruise to the Bahamas for what they spent on that damn dog." "Think of all the starving children they could have fed with that money. It makes me sick."

It didn't matter what guests thought; it made the owners feel good to know they had done everything possible for their pet. That included having Blackie bathed and trimmed at the funeral parlor before his viewing. "He looked his best," his owner told me, "very handsome." Price didn't matter.

In my day a standard bare-bones funeral in North Carolina ranged from $35 to $130 while a formal or more elaborate one cost $450 to $2500. These prices didn't necessarily include optional upgrades. For example, if you wanted the sturdier casket, it cost more. If you wanted the larger granite headstone or one with beveled edges, you paid more. If you had a large pet, it ran higher. Dog-Gone Owners, many of them dazed, vulnerable and distraught, paid the high price they had to to lay their pets and their minds to rest.

"Hey, I've seen memorial markers advertised in mail-order catalogues for $10.95," a client told me. "I could have ordered one for Little Lulu, instead of forking over a mint like I did. But that was no time to be chintzy. Hell, the funeral director could have asked me to sign over my house, and I would have."

Times haven't changed that much. The only exception is that a funeral costs more these days, and of course varies state to state. Currently, a Florida standard version runs around $475 and up, headstone not included, while the formal begins at about $925, including the generic granite headstone. Naturally, you pay more to upgrade the headstone to a carved heart, one with beveled borders or the larger-than-a-chair size. Standard or formal, there's an annual maintenance fee for the plot of around $40.00. You can add on today's inflated prices for catered food, flowers and liquor if you invite people back to your house after the ceremony.

The owner of a Florida establishment, a beautiful pet cemetery in a semi-rural area, offers a "country burial." This plan is ideal for the dog that doesn't need pomp and circumstance to get to that kennel in the sky or for an owner on a limited budget.

"It was a salve to my heart and pocketbook," one of my neighbors told me. For $150 her dog's body was picked up at the veterinarian's, delivered to the cemetery and buried in a lovely grassy and treed area. Since dogs are not embalmed, and since there was no casket, no viewing and no service, the price was minimal when you consider funerals. "I spent $10 more to have a small brass marker with Wolf's name placed on the memorial board," she said, "but that was it." This woman often visits her pet, and feels comfortable with her decision. "Wolf wasn't a fancy dog. He wasn't the kind of dog you dressed up or fed delicacies to or pampered. He was down to earth and loved the simple life. This is where he belongs," she told me with a smile.

There isn't a significant difference when you compare dog and people funerals. There are as many decisions to make for a pet as a person, and survivors suffer intensely through either. It's simply death on a smaller scale and at less cost, unless you're talking about some Dog-Gone Owners.

When I put myself in their place, and that is just about the last place I want to be, I choose to say goodbye to my pets in a private way, at home and in back yard burials. Going by experience, I'm not up to funeral planning when I'm devastated with grief. Apparently this doesn't hold true for many others who have lost pets. Every detail is worked out, and every one is important. Far from being a rarity, a pet funeral is commonplace, and generally adheres to the cultural or religious bent of the owner.

I attended an Irish wake for Shamus, a collie. The one night observance was held at the dog's home where many of his human relatives and friends walked up to the open casket in the living room to say goodbye to him. There was an abundance of food and liquor, singing and Shamus-related stories, and much laughter and tears. "How he would have loved this night," his smiling owner told me. "We sang his favorite songs, and everyone he loved had something good to say to him. He'll be happy when we lay him to rest tomorrow morning."

I attended the send-off for Desiree, a Lhasa Apso who died of congestive heart failure in her sleep when she was 14 1/2 years old. After her death, her owners took her home. Many friends, including some with dogs that wore black ribbons came to bid Desiree farewell.

Under different circumstances it would have been hilarious. Here were the owners trying to lead the dogs to the coffin to pay their respects. "Be a good boy, Spot and don't embarrass Momma!" And there were the dogs, tugging and scrambling to get in the opposite direction. "Wow, is that food in the bowls on the floor for me?" "Hey, I smell a female beagle!" I overheard one irate gentleman say to his Yorkie, "George, this is no time to be an ass sniffer!"

The next day, an inter-denominational service was held in a people chapel. Desiree's "uncle" was the funeral director there, and he would have done anything to help his sister and brother-in-law in their hour of need.

Bordered by large framed pictures of herself, Desiree was in an open casket where people could view her body. A sea of tears were shed by guests as they listened to the somber organ music softly wafting through the room, and the minister and close friends deliver eulogies. (See illustration 30.)

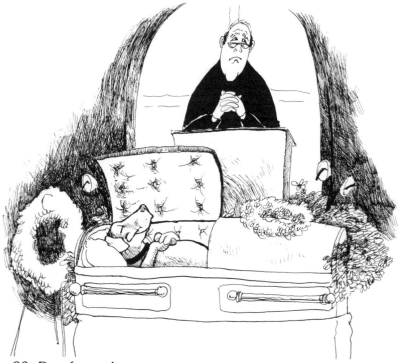

30. Dog funeral

After the service, Desiree's casket was closed and she was transferred to a hearse. We piled into our cars and followed the hearse to the pet cemetery. As the casket was lowered into the ground, her mistress had to be revived with smelling salts.

But the ordeal was worth it to her. It is to many owners.

Six to 20 owners a month arrange funerals with one local pet establishment. This in no way reflects the vast number of mourners as some owners leave the remains with the veterinarian and then return home to grieve, while others have private services at meaningful places.

Nor does this number reflect the number of dogs that are buried in people cemeteries in the same casket with their owners. It is possible to be buried with your pet. It is legal and possible to be buried with your pet, although it's not advertised. But that doesn't mean you can bring your pet to Tri-County Funeral Home or Shalom Memorial Gardens, or any place you've chosen for your personal resting place, have your pet interred, and then join him later. You have to accompany him.

How is that possible? An undertaker friend told me that many dogs are put to sleep immediately after the master or mistress's death so they can be buried together. "If the person specifies this in his or her will, it's done." He had performed this service many times, "more often than you'd think. I recently buried a woman with her Pekingese. She got the idea from her dead husband who had stated in his will that he wanted to be buried sitting in the driver's seat of his antique automobile. We did it."

An alternative is cremation. It was and still is less costly than burial, with the price ranging from $150 for small dogs like teacup poodles to $300 for Great Danes . . . and that's if you take the ashes home in an urn. The price increases if you want to bury the urn in a memorial garden and have a headstone, or place the urn in a wall niche with a bronze plaque.

"Mind you, I loved my dog," Melanie said. "Not as much as my husband loved the mutt, but I loved him enough to agree to have him cremated though we can afford that as much as we can afford to redo our living room, which we can't." They decided on cremation because her husband was claustrophobic, and the thought of burying Scooter made him feel like he was suffocating. "How could she breathe boxed in a coffin that's under tons of dirt?"

When asked why they decided to cremate pets, owners provided several reasons. "We're moving and want to take her with us. We can't abandon her." But, no matter what the reasons, they are all tied to the heart strings.

"Laddie loved to travel with us in the car. So we're going to leave a little bit of him in every state we visited," one woman told me. "He'd like that."

"We gave some of his ashes to our son and our daughter who are both married and live out of state, and we kept the rest. Everyone who loved him has part of him."

In this case, the daughter later told me she wasn't thrilled when her parents mailed her a gift-wrapped box containing one third of incinerated Imp. "How could I refuse it when Mom and Dad were crying like babies, and thought Imp's remains meant the same to me as it did to them? Now Imp makes a fast trip to the coffee table whenever my parents are due to arrive."

"My wife and I can't agree," one man told me. "I want Dudley to be on the fireplace mantle in my den. That's the room he slept in at nights. The wife wants him under our waterbed where he took his naps." They tried both places. When Dudley was in the bedroom, the husband dreamed he heard him crying. When he was in the den, the wife swore she heard him scratching on the door. "He wasn't at peace because we weren't." They settled the issue by buying a second urn and transferring half of Dudley into it so he could be in both rooms at once. "He's fine now, and so are we."

Bronze, wooden, brass, ceramic, onyx, you name it. You can have any urn you want as long as you pay for it. On the other hand, a few of my clients didn't invest in an urn. They couldn't bring the ashes home or dispose of them because that was too painful for them. Therefore, the funeral director disposed of the cremains, and the owners went home empty handed. "When Sylvester died, he died," one owner commented. "We have our memories; we don't need an urn to look at every day. That would be more than we could bear."

Another owner felt differently. "The wife and I couldn't stand the thought of deserting Sammy at the vet's or bringing him home. Sammy was a nature lover who reveled in being outdoors." This couple considered every option before narrowing them down to two: burying Sammy's urn in the cemetery garden or placing it in a niche in the memorial wall. "He's in the niche. It was a good compromise for him and us. He's outside where he loved to be, and we can talk to him without bending over and breaking our backs."

While many owners opted for urns, others used containers that had significance to them, such as: "This was the vase I bought for our first house the same day we adopted Basil." Another woman found a music box that played her dog's favorite song.

By far, the most creative idea came from a couple who managed to have their cremated dog blend in with their kitchen decor. They placed his ashes in his glass feeding bowl, and then had the bowl encased in Lucite. Not content with merely having Arf's initials monogrammed on one side, his owners had the Lucite etched with the saga, "Here lie the ashes of Arf Pitosky, who died a tragic death September 19, 1979, at the young age of 11 years and three months. God love you and watch over you, Arf. Love, Mommy and Daddy." Lucky for them, Arf was a Great Dane who used a large bowl.

While dog burial works for some people, and cremation works for others, there are Dog-Gone Owners who aren't content with either because you can't see the dog when it's under ground, and you can't pet ashes. But, there is one way to have a dead dog that still keeps your company.

Miss Murphy, a single woman who adored her dog, made an appointment to bring Piglet the pug to visit me. That was puzzling as Piglet had died three months previously. Thinking logically, it didn't make sense that I could see a dog that was dead. As it turned out, and not for the first time in my practice, logic was meaningless.

I walked into the examination room where Miss Murphy was talking into a pet carrier on the table.

"You have to see Piglet," she said. "Come on out, Baby." She opened the carrier door and pulled out the pug. "Isn't he beautiful?"

Indeed he was. His coat looked shiny and smooth, his nose looked wet and his eyes were bright. He looked wonderful, except he wasn't moving.

"I took you to a taxidermist, didn't I, you little angel," she crooned to the stuffed dog. She patted him. I patted him, too. We spent a few minutes admiring Piglet and then Miss Murphy put him back inside the carrier, and headed for the exit. "It's much easier now," she told me. "I don't have to walk him or feed him, and I'll have him around for the rest of my life." She walked out, talking to Piglet and telling him he was going for a ride in the car.

"That's a little abnormal, don't you think?" asked Abby, my assistant, who most definitely was not a Dog-Gone Owner. "I mean, maybe she needs psychiatric help, talking to a dead animal and having him stuffed, and all."

I thought about that for a little while before I answered, "No, I don't agree." I meant it.

Hunters have trophies of stuffed heads or full bodies of animals they've killed. Fishermen also have trophies of the big ones that didn't get away. As far as I know, they're for show, proof of the person's prowess. That's considered perfectly all right.

Why not stuff Piglet, and other domestic animals, who have for many years brought happiness and love to their owners? Taxidermy is one way that ensures togetherness. A person like Miss Murphy who was elderly didn't have to worry about leaving her money to heirs as she lacked family. By making the investment to stuff Piglet she had a constant companion.

To our way of thinking it might sound a little unusual, but Piglet was still alive to her although she realized he was dead. She talked to him, complained to him, laughed and cried to him and probably asked his advice. He filled a huge void in her life, and having him around made her a happy woman.

"But she talks to him," Abby repeated. Well, I told her, plenty of people talk to themselves. I do it often. And when I'm angry, I sometimes yell at people who aren't there. I also talk to my car, especially when it won't start or konks out in the middle of nowhere.

"And she takes him for rides?"

"Yes, and she said she'll keep on sleeping with him, too."

She is still sleeping with him. Today Miss Murphy is with Piglet in the hereafter. Her request that they be buried together was honored.

The beauty of taxidermy is that the pet can be immobilized in any position the owner desires. Piglet was "awake," stretched out on his tummy with his face on his paws. Another client's dog was in the same position, with closed eyes. He spent the next years in his favorite chair in the den, and nobody was allowed to move him to make room for themselves. Other dogs have been stuffed so they sit, stand and point, stand up and beg, or have fangs bared and look ready to attack. The owners usually chose the position they thought was the cutest or most realistic, or one they or the dog favored.

The one I liked best was the male setter with a raised hind leg. His master, who liked to fool around with electronics and gadgets, rigged a Rube Goldberg creation so that the dog peed onto a fire-hydrant that captured and recirculated the "urine." This might not be what you'd like to see in your front hallway, but the guy loved it. His wife was as delighted as the wife who endured the sight of her stuffed setter cleaning the private parts of his body. "Well, Hell," said that husband, "that's what he spent most of his days doing."

Taxidermy isn't for everyone but chances are more than one person in your town would have their spouse stuffed if that were legal. Mrs. North felt that way. "I couldn't take Mortimer to the taxidermist but I could and did take Custard. Why don't they let you stuff husbands?" Had she had her way, she said, Mortimer would be reading the paper in the living room, sitting in his chair, wearing boxer shorts and an undershirt. "Actually," she confided, "he liked to sit around in the buff but that would be too shocking for my friends to see."

I found Custard, a huge German Shepherd, cooling off in the bathtub. That's where he actually spent his stuffed years. "I have a shower stall, too, so I never have to disturb him," Mrs. North said. "I just cover his eyes before I undress to shower."

But, a word of caution to those of you who own more than one pet. Taxidermy might not be the way to go.

One client no sooner recovered from the shock of losing Rosie, one of her two cockapoos, and bringing her home from the taxidermist's, when she called me at home. "I'm scared out of my mind. I think Button is having a nervous breakdown. He's shivering and hiding under the bed and in the closets. I don't know what to do and I've tried everything I can think of.''

I made a house call. Button didn't come when his mistress called him. He didn't come when I called him, either, and that was unusual because the cockapoo used to trip over his feet running to greet me in the clinic. We finally cajoled him out of a closet, and he accompanied us to the dining room, but he absolutely refused to follow us into the living room. He stood at the doorway and shook like crazy.

I glanced into the room and there was Rosie, looking as if she were taking a nap on the fireplace mantel-piece. Button's eyes were riveted on his stuffed ex-buddy. I approached Rosie, and Button began to howl and shake even more. Evidently, he knew the difference between a live pal and a dead one, and he didn't appreciate seeing stiff and quiet Rosie lying there. He made a fast and complete recovery when Rosie was moved to a closet shelf.

It was an expensive experience for this owner. As taxidermy prices are high, depending on the size of the animal. Today, taxidermists have a machine that freeze-dries creatures, preserving them almost perfectly, with each hair as it was. These prices range from $300 to $500 for a small dog and $1000 to $1200 for a large one, again with prices varying state to state.

In my practicing days it ran about $100 to stuff a small dog and $200 to $300 for a large one. Even then, when costs were less, I couldn't understand why one client had her dog stuffed and then buried. That impressed me as a rather extreme measure. Why do both when one does the job? Curiosity got the better of me until I asked the owner why she had done both.

"It was Watusi's blanket,'' she said. Evidently, after Watusi was stuffed, her owners thought she'd be more comfortable if they covered her with her favorite blanket each evening. All was fine until the grandchildren visited. "They wouldn't leave Watusi's blanket alone. They kept grabbing it and running around the house like Batman. I can't tell you how this disturbed our doggy. To give her peace, we buried her with her blanket." I told her that was a very sensible solution. "Maybe so, but she misses us. We have to go to the cemetery to visit her, and she hates it when we leave."

Now we're in the era of cyrogenics, freezing people or just the heads of people, and storing the part or parts in cylinders that are maintained at a constant temperature. The thinking is that someday they can be revived and rejoin their loved ones on earth. Unfortunately, by the time scientists perfect this art it's doubtful many familiar people will be around to greet them. "That's beside the point," Mrs. Young told me. "You either believe, or you don't believe."

Most of us don't believe. The idea seems ludicrous, insane or too remote. I realize it is reasonable however, to someone like my distant cousin who abandoned everyday life to live in India learning about past lives and reincarnation. And to people like Mrs. Young.

Mr. Young was frozen. Mrs. Young plans to be. It was natural that she chose this option for her chow.

"Even if it hadn't been in Ming's will I still would have done it," she told me. "Unless, of course, he had reconsidered." Wiping away her tears, she added, "It's comforting beyond words to know we'll all be sitting together around the breakfast table again some year."

Speaking of wills brings up another facet of dying, death and disposition. A few of my clients made sure their dogs had their own documents. As I previously mentioned, it's highly unusual for Dog-Gone Owners to face the issue of their dogs' death, but as in everything there's an exception to the rule.

"It was a necessity," insisted Emily and Fred. "We're not as young as we used to be. What if we die before Jet? Who will grant his final wishes?"

They had their children over for a family meeting. Jet was included, and told the purpose of the get-together was to make sure he had a say in his fate. When I asked how the dog communicated what he wanted, I was informed that it was easier than it sounds.

"We sat Jet down and went through the list of options. You know, like burial or cremation? Back yard or cemetery? With or without toys? Things like that. He barked to let us know. Then we went on to each possession, and asked him which of his friends he wanted to remember with his clothes and toys and other possessions. We even discussed his stone, and he told us he wants a metal photo of himself attached to a gray granite headstone."

After this, Emily typed up the will, and Jet "signed" it with his paw print as two neighbors witnessed his signature. The children swore on their lives they'd abide by Jet's wishes if their parents preceded him in death, and Fred added the will to the other important papers in their safety deposit box at the bank.

"Nobody likes to think of dying," Fred remarked. "It wasn't until last year that Emily could discuss anyone's death. She'd always start to cry and tell me we could talk about it later. Then Pepe, the dog next door, died suddenly and we realized death could happen any time. That's why we had Jet write his will. We'll get around to ours when we have the time."

As the saying goes, first things first. Obviously, it's more important to think of the pet's death. And as a client said, "When a pet dies, it stinks."

It does. It hurts terribly. It's tremendous painful to know you'll never again see your pet, or laugh about something funny or cute he just did, or feel that loving and wonderfully soft body against yours.

That's under the best of circumstances, when you have a support system of understanding people who appreciate what you're going through and share your pain. But what do you do when you feel alone and have nobody by your side?

"I left the SOB," Reba told me. "We had been married less than a year and were supposedly still on our honeymoon. But when Pupsky died, I discovered my husband was incapable of showing an ounce of compassion. He told me I was immature when I asked for a hug or cried as I looked at photos of Pupsky. I moved in with a dog-loving girlfriend."

"I called my veterinarian frequently," another owner contributed. "I was at his clinic when a woman brought in her dog that had been killed by a car a few minutes before. I knew he'd treat me with dignity after my dog died, too."

Fortunately, veterinarians are naturally compassionate souls with a good bedside manner and a love of animals. Some cry with you. Others let you know that without doubt their sympathy is with you. They're trained to give advice when a pet is dying or has died, and let you know your options.

"I'm so happy you told me about pet funerals," Mrs. Garver told me. "I didn't know they existed. The woman there was wonderful. She was like a bereavement counselor and understood what I was going through. She helped me accept Winky's death."

Sooner or later, most grieving owners do accept it. Some manage with time, others with a little help or change of scenery, and a few with doses of intense therapy.

A handful of Dog-Gone Owners confided that they needed private sessions with a psychiatrist. One woman in an unhappy marriage, said, "It was expensive but rewarding. At home I had to be strong or my husband yelled. Through therapy I had a safe haven for a couple of hours every week. I could be myself, and not have someone tell me I was acting foolish or crazy before walking out in a huff."

"My lifesaver was attending a pet loss and grieving support group," said another, this one an unmarried career woman. "How many people know that the Humane Society offers this? I went for months, just to cry and talk about Lancelot with other people in my shoes. I didn't have to cover up my feelings; I could let it all hang out and nobody thought I was over-emotional or ridiculous.

"Now," she said, "I've found closure. I remember Lancelot alive, and how happy he was to be with me. I don't need his body because his spirit is with me, around me, always. Instead of mourning his death, I can genuinely celebrate that I had him as long as I did."

A good friend of mine, Ina Forbus, wrote the following poem for her four Scotties.

> Dear God, I ask for these small friends
> A wide green path for eager feet
> That daily raced on cool green grass
> And were not used to city streets.
> And could You please give them a creek
> Around the bend of which adventure lie
> And let them chase a rabbit up the hill and down;
> They'll never catch him but it's fun to try.
> Just one more thing, Dear Father, I would ask:
> LET ME BE GREETED AT THE OUTER DOOR
> BY ALL THE MADLY WAGGING TAILS AND
> LOVING EYES OF MY DEAR FOUR.

May all the departed dogs continue to rest in peace. They were lucky pets to have been loved so deeply by their owners.

Chapter 11

And The Award Goes To . . . !

I believe the majority of veterinarians primarily chose the profession because of their love of animals, and their intense desire to heal them and to be around them. But equally important and definitely welcome is the contact these doctors have with their patients' owners. As one colleague told me, "I need to see and talk to clients, too. Although I love my patients, some of my best friends are people."

All veterinarians have a special place in their hearts or memories for special clients who, for one reason or another, stand out from the thousands of other. Here are a few of my Dog-Gone winners.

THE AWARD FOR MOST EXPENSIVE AND EXTENSIVE MANICURE AND PEDICURE goes to Mrs. Abernathy. Mrs. A. brought her poodle, Dipsy Doodle, into the clinic 16 times and hired 16 taxis to have her dog's nails clipped for one manicure/pedicure! "It would be too much of a shock to her nervous system to have them clipped one after the other," Mrs. A. said. "She'd be devastated for life." So, she arranged to have me clip one nail a day. That comes to sixteen sessions and 16 taxi fares. Plus tips. Now multiply this by three or four times to arrive at her annual investment. (See Illustration 31)

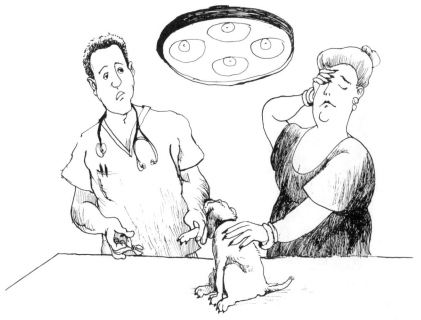

31. One nail at a time!

The BOSOM BUDDY AWARD goes to Babette Brown. Mrs. B.'s epic bust size would put Dolly Parton to shame. While Mrs. B. didn't believe in the adage, "If you have it, flaunt it," she found her bosom came in handy for her Chihuahua that was susceptible to chills and drafts. Mrs. B. kept

ChiChi warm and cozy by toting her around town and to dog shows tucked in her ample cleavage. (See Illustration 32)

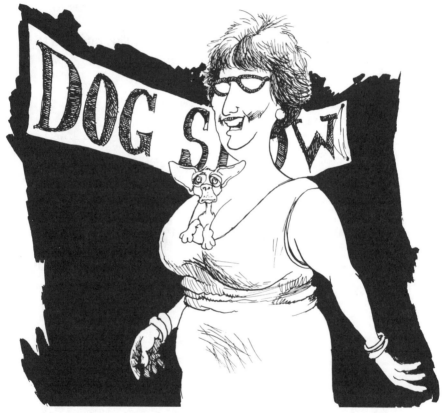

32. Bosom carrier

The CHEAPER BY THE DOZEN AWARD goes to Mrs. Trueheart. Mrs. T's Pekingese was an angel. "His only bad habit," she said, "is urinating on a woman's legs if she's wearing stockings. Not one of her legs, but both." Mrs. T. tried in vain to break Peekie of this annoying habit. "It was costing me a fortune to replace brand name nylons for my friends. After all, I had to do something to show them I sincerely regretted my dog's actions besides apologize." Finally, Mrs. T. bought dozens of pairs of nylon stockings in varying shades and sizes at a discount outlet. "Then, when Peekie turned on his faucet, which was constant, I immediately fetched the basket filled with stockings and let my friends pick out a pair or two. That immediately appeased them."

The IT'S THE THOUGHT, NOT THE GIFT THAT COUNTS AWARD goes to wealthy and generous Mrs. Conway. Mrs. C. honored me in her will by bequeathing me her 29 dogs, even though I had informed her beforehand that unlike her I would not sleep with any of them. Still, she knew I'd do a dandy job of ensuring that her babies thrived under my care. They did, although the dogs were all endowed with long lives, and the lady neglected to allocate any money to me for their upkeep. (See illustration 33)

The CRY WOLF or "Oh, no, not that woman again award," goes to Minnie McAnn. Minnie was a woman who tried to drown her problems in alcohol. When she became intoxicated, at least two or three times each month, usually in the middle of the night, she'd call me. "Lou, I'm going to kill myself and I want you to promise to take care of Mutt and Jeff."

Each time Minnie phoned, it took me 20 to 30 minutes to convince her that she couldn't do away with herself as no one else in the world could or would take as good care of her dogs

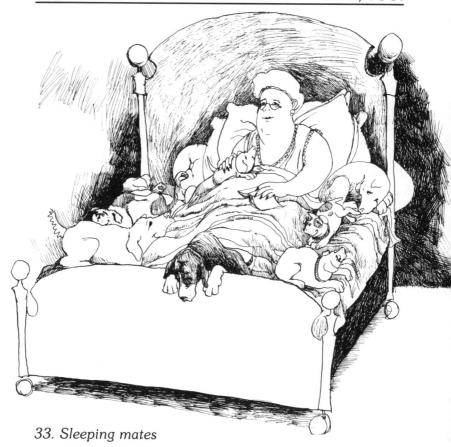

33. Sleeping mates

as she. She was necessary and vital to their welfare. Still the calls continued.

As Minnie had told me the name of her psychiatrist, I consulted him , and he assured me I was using the correct approach. Evidently he was right as Minnie snapped out of each suicidal threat until her next binge. (See illustration 34)

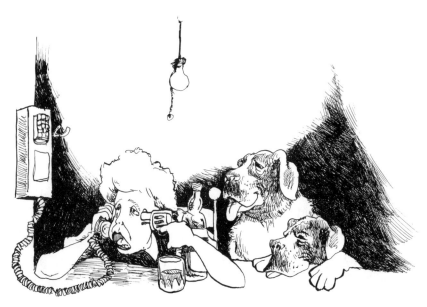

34. Saving a life

The SETTLE FOR LESS AWARD goes to Ducky and Regis Parker. Their Great Dane insisted on sleeping in the master bedroom on the king-sized bed. "He slept with us from the time he was a puppy. He's big now, and he hates it when we get into bed and wake him from a sound sleep." Sultan hated it so much he began to growl and bare his fangs. "No problem, now," they told me. "We moved into the guest room."

The DANDY DECISION AWARD goes to Dan Devan. Like most dogs, Dan's dog loved to ride in the car and feel the wind in his face. Unlike most dogs, O'Toole would not take no for an answer; he'd beg and howl until he got his wish. It wasn't always convenient for Dan to cruise around town with his dog, but he had an alternative plan. He'd put O'Toole in the car, open the car windows, direct a large floor fan toward a window, and turn it on full blast in the dog's face. O'Toole was delighted and satisfied, and so was Dan, except when he received his monthly electric bill. But, look at all the gasoline money he saved.

The FIRST THINGS FIRST AWARD goes to an heiress worth millions who willed her estate to the state veterinary college research fund. The only hitch was that until her dog died, the college couldn't touch a penny. Years passed before the university collected its due, minus the money that had been spent keeping the dog in the lavish lifestyle to which he was accustomed.

The MASTER OF INGENUITY AWARD goes to Fred Franklin. No one could bathe his Saint Bernard. Fred couldn't do it alone, and he couldn't do it with the assistance of three friends. Buck would take one look at people approaching him, knew they'd try to lure him into the bathtub, and he'd go into an attack mode, biting anything or anyone he could get his teeth into. After I declined the privilege of accepting the challenge, and Buck was smelling quite ripe, Fred hit on the solution. "He gets his bath every month now, and loves it. I can't believe it's the same dog." Fred changed into a bathing suit and took his dog for a ride in his convertible. "With the top down, we go through the car wash." No, it didn't hurt the leather interior of the car. "From the carwash, I drive Buck home and then have the car detailed. You know, cleaned, vacuumed and buffed from top to bottom, inside and out."

The BIGGEST PAIN IN THE BUTT AWARD goes to the woman who refused to spay her dog or keep her locked in the house when she was in heat. "Neutering is brutal and inhuman," she'd tell me. When the dog got pregnant and went into labor, twice a year, she'd called me in the middle of the night, to ask," Are you home?"

"I think I am. Why?"

"Eloise is in labor."

"Is she having trouble?"

"No. But I wanted to find out if you're home in case we need you."

Through more litters and years than I can count, Eloise managed on her own.

The MRS. FASTIDIOUS AWARD goes to Mrs. Johnson who would not allow her poodle to go outside for "walkies" for fear Dixie would pick up fleas, get her feet wet or lose her virginity to the altered Doberman next door. Instead, Mrs. Johnson spread papers on the bathroom floor and invested a considerable amount of time in that room potty training Dixie.

Predictably, Dixie learned to associate evacuating with her audience, and produced only when her mistress was there to watch and to praise her. Then, she'd jump up on the closed toilet seat and whine until Mrs. Johnson wiped her bottom. Mrs. Johnson was considering the feasibility of buying a bidet for her dog. "I don't know what to do," she said. "I'm sure it would make her more squeaky clean, but I don't want Dixie to develop an anal fixation." (See illustration 35)

The TRUE LOVE AWARD goes to a woman who came to my clinic with her four year old son and five year old dog. While they were in the waiting room, the little boy began to cry.

"Stop it," the mother ordered. When he didn't, she slapped him with the dog's leash. He cried harder. 'Behave yourself

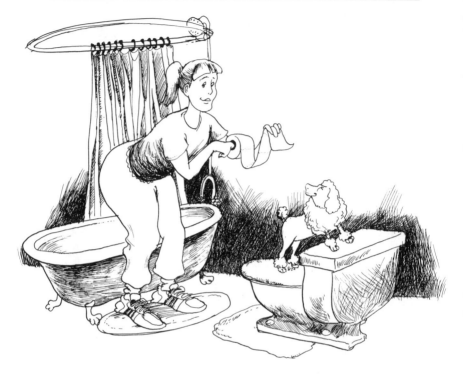

35. Toilet service

and shut up! I've had this dog longer than I've had you, and I can get rid of you.''

"Mommy,'' the little boy sobbed, ''you love the dog more than you love me.''

Mother answered, ''You bet I do.''

The UNEXPECTED BENEFIT AWARD goes to Mrs. Wayne, a long-time widow, who put an ad in a newspaper for a canine pen pal for her dog. ''Fernando was lonely and needed to hear from friends,'' she explained. Within a few months, Fernando had received enough replies from people and their dogs to give the mailman a backache. "I read Fernando every card and letter that arrives, Mrs. Wayne said, "and some days that can take hours and hours." Before Christmas, Mrs. Wayne sent a card in Fernando's name to each dog on the pen pal list. And then some of the owners started writing to her as well as Fernando. One turned out to be a local Dog-Gone widower who complimented her on her devotion to her pet. They "introduced" their dogs at a nearby park, and shortly after this, the owners married. All four went on the honeymoon. (See illustration 36)

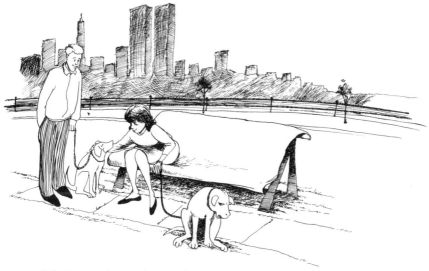

36. Penpals in the park

The THIS, TOO, SHALL PASS AWARD goes to Alicia Peachtree. Alicia wanted a diamond collar for her Russian Wolfhound. "He just had to have one."

As you know, diamonds are less expensive overseas, so whenever Alicia and Noble traveled, Alicia purchased a couple of them. Not wanting to pay duty, "we both swallowed a small one before we boarded the plane back to the U.S.." This system worked for quite a few trips. "But we still needed an extra large diamond for the center of the collar before the jeweler could begin to create it."

Shortly after they returned from Europe, Alicia went to the hospital complaining of a fierce stomach ache. The doctor diagnosed an acute intestinal blockage, and recommended surgery. When he operated, he spotted a diamond that was caught in a loop of Alicia's small intestine. It cost Alicia a fortune in medical and surgical bills, but Noble got his collar with the spectacular diamond, and became the talk of the town.

Epilogue

At the beginning of my practice, when I started collecting facts and histories, I thought Dog-Gone Owners were excessively enthusiastic in some of the ways they related to their pets. But as I started to write this book, and as it progressed, I saw more of myself in each chapter.

Doggone it, I'm a Dog-Gone Owner, too. I've been one all along, and never knew it. And I'm proud to be one.

I like to think that I'm not as extreme as some of the people I've mentioned, but if you were to ask my wife, she'd tell you I'm at the head of the line. "Why else, Lou, have you always told clients and audiences that came to your lectures that there's nothing wrong with spoiling anyone you love, be it person or dog, as long as you don't overdo it? Dog-Gone Owners overdo it. So do you, dear."

But, before I knew I was one, I learned a lot from my kindred souls. They showed me the meaning of unconditional love and total devotion. I talk about it, the more dedicated Dog-Gone Owners live it as they share life with their pets. They're like my friend who won't wear eyeglasses because without them everyone is beautiful and has no flaws.

225

My thanks go to my Dog-Gone friends. They kept me on my toes for 40 years, delighted me, aggravated me, surprised me, shocked me and excited me. Without them, my veterinary career would have been nothing but fur and feathers. With them, and because of their "unusual" beliefs and actions, it was a joy.